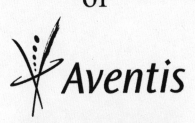

"A book filled with what I call 'survival behavior.' A meaningful life is built on love and laughter, and this book shares both and shows us where to find them in our lives. I recommend it to all those who have the desire to be survivors. The treatment of cancer has side effects just as cancer does. Read this and learn that all the side effects are not negative ones."

—Bernie Siegel, M.D., author of *Love, Medicine and Miracles* and *Prescriptions for Living*

"The perfect dose of medicine for anyone whose life has been touched by cancer. After reading this book, it is obvious that those who battle cancer are the true gold medal winners of life."

—Michele Smith, two-time Olympic gold medallist, Women's Softball, Pitcher

"[This book] can help you find joy in difficult times. You'll smile and laugh aloud as you read this collection of entertaining stories. More important, Christine Clifford encourages you to find and enjoy the humor in your own life. When you can let the humor arise from within, you can feel good every day." —Wendy S. Harpham, M.D., author of *After Cancer. A Guide to Your New Life* and *When a Parent Has Cancer. A Guide to Caring for Your Children*

"Christine Clifford has a gift for blending powerful insights with heartwarming stories and practical advice. Funny, profound, reassuring and inspiring. A must-read for anyone coping with cancer."

—Elise NeeDell Babcock, author of *When Life Becomes Precious;* founder of Cancer Counseling, Inc.

"You don't have to have had cancer to be a survivor. Christine's inspirational and pathologically positive attitude should be shared by everyone who has faced adversity. God definitely has a plan for this woman."

—Larry Gatlin, Grammy Award®–winning singer/songwriter

"I heartily recommend *Cancer Has Its Privileges* as a delightful addition to the library of any cancer survivor. Everyone talks about the war on cancer, but this book can certainly provide laughter between the battles."

—D. Lawrence Wickerham, M.D., associate chairman of the NSABP (National Surgical Adjuvant Breast and Bowel Project)

Praise for Christine Clifford:

"I've always felt that humor is better than chicken soup for the healing process . . . Christine Clifford handles a grave subject matter with sensitivity and warmth." —Jim Davis, cartoonist and creator of *Garfield*

"You are doing great work. I am inspired by your message."
—Jack Canfield, co-author of *Chicken Soup for the Soul*

"I have learned to laugh again and anew thanks to a wonderful friend by the name of Christine Clifford, who has prescribed for me God's great gift and healing powers of laughter."
—Dr. William H. Nace, United Methodist minister

Cancer Has Its Privileges:

Stories of Hope and Laughter

Christine Clifford

Illustrated by Jack Lindstrom

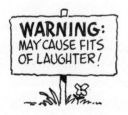

A PERIGEE BOOK

A Perigee Book
Published by The Berkley Publishing Group
A division of Penguin Putnam Inc.
375 Hudson Street
New York, New York 10014

First edition: May 2002

Visit our website at www.penguinputnam.com

LIBRARY OF CONGRESS CATALOGING-IN-PUBLICATION DATA

Clifford, Christine, 1954–
Cancer has its privileges : stories of hope and laughter / written by
Christine Clifford; illustrated by Jack Lindstrom.
p. cm.
Includes bibliographical references.
ISBN: 0-399-52776-1
1. Cancer—Popular works. 2. Cancer in women—Anecdotes. I. Title.

RC263 .C56 2002
362.1'96994'0082—dc21
2001058755

PRINTED IN THE UNITED STATES OF AMERICA
10 9 8 7 6 5

*To my husband, John, sons, Tim and Brooks,
and to all the family, friends and members of The Cancer Club®
who have helped make my life privileged.*

To the Memory of
*my mother, Mary Christine,
and to all our contributing authors
who are no longer with us today: Deborah Bauserman,
Edward Beckwell, Rita Busch, Linda Forti,
Mary Minor, Robert H. Mueller,
and Kris Silverman.*

Contents

Acknowledgments

You will find, as you look back upon your life,
that the moments that stand out are the moments
when you have done things for others.
—HENRY F. DRUMMOND

I could never begin to thank all the amazing people who
have done things for me in my journey with cancer. From little
things to big things, I believe that this particular aspect of my
cancer experience has been my greatest gift. To receive unconditional love, support, concern, humor, but most of all—friendship
has been the privilege of a lifetime.

I would like to thank the following individuals for helping me
make *Cancer Has Its Privileges: Stories of Hope and Laughter* a reality:

My beloved husband, John, whom I met my freshman year in
college and who has been my best friend for twenty-nine years.
My two boys, Tim and Brooks, who bring me joy and happiness
on a daily basis. I thank the three of them for being my foundation and greatest source of humor.

My extended family including sister Pam Meyer and brother-
in-law Nick Haros, my brothers Greg and James Meyer, my
mother-in-law Bette Clifford, my step-mother Stephanie Meyer,
my step-sister Kristin Bauersfeld (also a survivor!) and my brother-

in-law Bill Clifford. I thank them for surrounding me with love and encouragement.

My illustrator, Jack Lindstrom, who captured the essence of my being and for his generosity of spirit and heart; my agent, Jeanne Hanson, for "discovering" me in a sea of authors; my editor, Sheila Curry Oakes, and her assistant, Terri Hennessy, at Penguin Putnam for believing in me and my work. I thank them for supporting my vision.

My next-door neighbor Madonna Koenig for her endless administrative work on the book, my account executive Lynn Lufkin for keeping things humming in the office while I was off writing or speaking, and my "virtual" secretary Jill Peterson for staying on top of my paperwork. I thank these three women for their daily dedication.

My physicians, Dr. Margit L. Bretzke, Dr. Burton Schwartz, Dr. Tae Kim, Dr. James Gaviser, and Dr. Carol Featherstone, along with their staff and technicians for their superb ministry. I thank them for the gift of my life.

My members of The Cancer Club® who believe in the power of positive thinking and know that laughter is, indeed, the best medicine. I thank all of the contributing authors for sharing their stories, without which this book would not exist. I thank you all for your willing and gracious participation.

The thousands of friends, acquaintances, associates, and strangers who have helped me find true meaning in my life. Special thanks to: Dr. Clarence "Buck" Brown, Linda Kay Smith, Etta Erickson and Margie Sborov, Whitney and Nancy Peyton, Bill and Barb Winchell, the "girls who lunch" (Pat Miles, Virginia Carlson, Kathy Lewis and Julie Nelson), friends Paula Bergs, Mary Evans, Molly Gill-Ramczyk, Jeff Evans, and anyone who has put up with playing a round of golf with me. I thank you for your friendship.

My many volunteers, committee members and sponsors for The Christine Clifford Celebrity Golf Invitational who have given endless hours of time, services and donations to make our event such a phenomenal success. Special recognition to Dawn Dempsey, Dave and Jeanne Mooty, Ruth Donaldson, Barb Schultz, Dave Knoblauch, Gerald McCullagh and celebrities Amy Grant, Larry Gatlin, Cameron Mathison, Scott Thompson Baker, Kelly Leadbetter, Sherrin Smyers, and Paul Magers along with all of the celebrities who so generously give of their time and commitment. I thank you for teaching me the art of philanthropy.

But most of all, I would like to thank God for blessing me with good health, a strong faith, a loving family, an abundance of friends, a passion for creativity, a vision of purpose and the gift of life and laughter.

Laughter is the heart's way of giving thanksgiving. Thank you for being a part of my life.

Foreword

Just a very few years ago, a group of women in Orlando, Florida, raising money for the breast cancer programs at our center, invited a young breast cancer survivor to speak to the gathering and play in a golf tournament that was the focal point of their fund-raising efforts. As CEO of the Cancer Center, I was asked to greet this young woman and serve as her host. Thus began my friendship with one of the most inspiring persons whom I have had the privilege to meet in my nearly three decades of caring for cancer patients.

That young woman, Christine Clifford, has become an icon to men and women from every corner of this globe. She is a true spokesperson for those who have entered the arena of cancer, frightened of the potential that such a diagnosis brings, believing there is nothing but bleakness in their future. Christine has changed that view for thousands and thousands of men and women and their families through her incredible ability to make people laugh.

Cancer Has Its Privileges: Stories of Hope and Laughter, Christine's fourth book, is yet another of her "gifts" to us who have to battle cancer either as a patient, a loved one, or as one who metes out some of those awful treatments we hear so much about. She uncannily finds humor where most would not think it could be, and as we see in this marvelous book, she inspires others to do that as well.

If there is one "privilege" that cancer has brought me, not as a survivor, but rather as an oncologist, it has been the privilege of my becoming a friend to Chris Clifford. A regrettable void would have existed in my career had I never come to know this beautiful, boundlessly energetic, motivating, and very funny woman.

I know you will enjoy *Cancer Has Its Privileges: Stories of Hope and Laughter*. You will laugh, but mostly you will see the hope. Christine has seen to that once again.

CLARENCE H. BROWN, III, M.D.
PRESIDENT AND CHIEF EXECUTIVE OFFICER
M. D. ANDERSON CANCER CENTER, ORLANDO

Introduction

May you live all the days of your life.
—Jonathan Swift

*Like most of us who have fought and won the war against cancer,
Christine Clifford is still in the process of monitoring her treatments
and side effects, but she's winning her battle against cancer. In fact,
Christine immediately began focusing on helping other people look on
the bright side of their situation. Allow me to introduce you to a
remarkable woman whose sense of humor became her best weapon
against an often dehumanizing disease.*

Arnold Palmer

Every December 19th I celebrate my anniversary as a cancer survivor. As I reflect back on the many years and my cancer experience, I can honestly say I would never go back and change that experience.

When I was diagnosed with cancer in '94, I only had one objective: I wanted to live. If I lived, I knew that I desired to make some changes in my life that would give me more time with my family and friends, and find work that brought meaning to my life. I've been fortunate, blessed and yes—lucky—to have found those things with The Cancer Club®, the company I founded in 1995 to market humorous and helpful products for people with cancer.

But most of all, I knew that if I lived and found meaning in my life, that I wanted to become philanthropic—to give something back to others less fortunate than I.

Too often we spend too much time dwelling on our own situation. Often we can't change our situation—I can never go back and change the fact that I had cancer. But the one thing we can change and do something about is our "ATTITUDE," and how we choose to deal with that "situation" on a go-forward basis.

For me personally, cancer has been a gift. It has given me the unique opportunity in my lifetime, while I'm still here on earth, to feel the love and support of family, friends, caregivers, and complete strangers.

It has allowed me the opportunity to do creative things I never knew I had inside of me: write books, design cartoons, start my own business and travel the world speaking to others who are facing, fighting and surviving the disease.

It has renewed my faith and reminded me that it's better to give than to receive. It has opened my eyes to volunteer opportunities and challenged me to share the knowledge and experiences I've had in the hope that my efforts may benefit another.

It has brought joy and laughter into my life on a daily basis and connected me with all of you—the members of The Cancer Club®—who share a common bond that there can, indeed, be moments of humor in the midst of all of our challenges.

I can remember as a cancer patient how I lived for the mailbox every day. Just to receive a card, letter, note or call made me feel like I wasn't alone in this journey—that someone out there was thinking about me. The Cancer Club®, through its quarterly newsletter, has strengthened that bond and the communication between cancer patients all over the world.

The excerpts in this book are but a small collection of the stories, poetry and submissions that cancer patients have been sending me and The Cancer Club® all these years. I've spent these years laughing with all of you—the patients, survivors, family members, friends, caregivers and employers—about the mishaps, awkward situations, catastrophes and blunders that cancer brought our way. I hope that these stories and poems bring the joy and laughter into your life that they've brought into mine.

Luck, timing, prayers, friendships, support, hard work, laughter and high expectations are what have led me to this important milestone in the life of every cancer patient: the gift of life. I want to thank all of YOU for helping me to be a survivor.

Whether you are newly diagnosed, or a longtime survivor, your life will never be the same. It can be better and better with each and every day as we celebrate our lives and look for opportunities to share our experiences and spread the knowledge of what it takes to WIN!

It has been an honor and a privilege meeting so many coura-
geous, determined and humorous cancer patients who gave so
freely of their hearts and clearly demonstrated the resiliency of
the human spirit. Give a gift of time, knowledge or just support
to someone less fortunate than yourself. After all, we're here, and
it's a great day to be alive. Don't forget to laugh!™

CHAPTER I

Humor: The Last Thing on My Mind

Laughter may not always add years to your life,
but it will add life to your years.
—AUTHOR UNKNOWN

"I have a black cat who shows absolutely no affection most of the time.
Four years ago, during my first battle with cancer, when my hair came
out, she slept curled around my head. Now I thought she did this
because she finally loved me. Imagine my pain when my husband
assured me it was for her own warmth! I'm on
chemo again, and she doesn't come near my
head, so he must be right. The house is a lot
warmer this go-around."
DONNA MALONEY, EL PASO, TEXAS

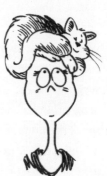

I had always enjoyed a good laugh, but it wasn't until I was diagnosed with breast cancer eight years ago that I realized how important my sense of humor would become in my fight against this disease. Today I am a veteran of the surgery, aggressive chemotherapy and radiation treatments that are commonplace to most cancer patients. But unlike most survivors, my strength comes from a unique perspective on the experience . . .

I was fifteen years old when my mother was diagnosed with breast cancer. The year was 1969. I'll never forget the day my father, a prestigious physician in the Los Angeles area, told me my mother was going to the hospital to have a lump removed.

In those days there were few choices when it came to cancer. At the age of thirty-eight, my mother woke up after surgery to discover she'd undergone a radical mastectomy.

Life had never been easy for my mother. Of her four children, two boys and two girls, my youngest brother was born with a congenital kidney defect and had undergone twenty-three major surgeries before the age of five. My older brother developed a drug problem in high school that required extensive electric shock therapy, the treatment of choice in the early 60s.

Quiet and introverted, my mother quickly sank into a deep depression after the mastectomy. She never pulled out of it.

Nowadays we have more effective treatments for clinical depression than there were in the 1960s. My mother was put on medication that left her helpless to cope with everyday living. She stopped washing her hair or brushing her teeth. She hardly ever left her bed in the months—then years—that followed her surgery.

After a while my father, unable to cope with my mother's behavior, moved out and separated from her. His leaving deepened her despair. When I graduated from high school and left for college, all I could think about was how happy I was to get away, to start pursuing a life of academia, sports, friendship and causes.

I'd only been gone for three months when I flew home from Colorado to California for Thanksgiving. When I walked into my mother's room, her usual place of rest, I noticed with horror that her remaining breast seemed unusually large through the sheer fabric of her nightgown.

I immediately got her dressed and loaded her into my car. It wasn't difficult. She was a tiny woman of barely 100 pounds. I drove to my father's clinic. As I sat in the examining room with my mother on the table, her blouse was slowly removed to reveal a breast that had become severely metastasized, possible over several years. She was taken directly to the hospital, where a second mastectomy was performed at once.

My mother died in May of that year, at the age of forty-two. I was holding her hand when she took her last breath. At that moment I prayed to God that no matter what He had in store for me in the years ahead, I wouldn't be confronted with cancer.

The year I turned forty, I had just come off the most successful year of my career as senior executive vice president of an international marketing company. My husband and I were buying a new house. We had two healthy, active boys, Tim, eleven, and Brooks, eight. We were coming up on our twentieth wedding anniversary. Life was great! It came to a screeching halt in a day.

I found a lump in my breast during a routine self-exam. While three different doctors told me it probably wasn't cancerous, I finally talked my gynecologist into doing a needle biopsy. Four days later my fears were confirmed, and I was scheduled for surgery on New Year's Eve.

One Wednesday

"Cancer," you say . . .
"That's quite a shock."
Should I cry?
Or Scream?
Or just take a walk?
Some cells in my body
Are on a grim march
And the news
Leaves me limp
Skin
With no starch.

My bones instantly
Seem to turn
Into jelly
A rumble of panic
Goes straight to
My belly.

As I am
About to implode
My surgeon calmly
Puts his hand on mine
And says,
"We can fight this.
Things can turn out just fine.

"It won't be easy.
Yet remember
You're strong.
And I'll do all I can
To help you along."

I believed what he said
With all of my heart
And that's how I got off
To a very good start.

DEBORAH TRENEER PITMAN, RICHLAND, WASHINGTON

I think back now in retrospect, that of all of the thousands of people I have met who have been told, "I'm so sorry. You have cancer," that I took the news harder than a freshly laid brick on the road that we call life. After all, my mother had been my role model. All I could think about was, "I'm going to get depressed, my husband will leave me, and I'll die." I remember thinking, "My life will never be the same, and I will never laugh again."

I can clearly remember the first time I laughed following my diagnosis. It was the day after Christmas and my husband, John, and I gathered our two boys in the family room to prepare them for the week ahead.

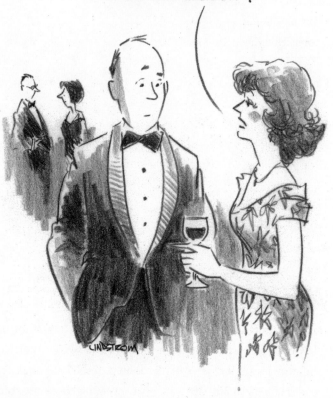

"Didn't we have a nice Christmas?" John asked, the boys squealing in delight at their haul of gifts and candies.

"Aren't we a lucky family?" he suggested with the boys nodding in unison at their small, charmed lives.

"Well, sometimes along with the good things, some bad things happen to people," he continued.

Pulling all of his second-grade frame to its full potential, Brooks pronounced, "Thank you for sharing that with us, Dad." John and I looked at each other and chuckled. "Your mom has a disease called cancer. She'll be going into the hospital this week for surgery. She's going to have some treatments that may cause her to become sick and lose her hair."

"Cool!" exclaimed Tim, his mind running wild with imagination. "You'll look like Captain Picard on *Star Trek*!"

I couldn't help but laugh. And I realized that that was the first time I had laughed in eight days.

It's true—our lives will never be the same. But that doesn't mean that we can't have a great life, a "new" life, a creative life, a life filled with love. As Amy Grant says, sometimes "it takes a little time sometime, to get your feet back on the ground."

We all will laugh again. Sometimes the impossible just takes a little bit longer . . .

CHAPTER II

Learning to Laugh Again

Learning to laugh at trouble radically increases
the amount of things there are to laugh at.
—AUTHOR UNKNOWN

"When I went for my presurgical visit for my gluteal flap, the plastic surgeon of course had five medical students (all good-looking young men) in tow. He was drawing in purple marker on my buttock. Here I am bare-assed on my stomach with six men looking at my rear! The surgeon was showing the students the major landmarks and said, 'First we locate the major dimple . . .' and I chimed out 'I'm sure there's more than one major dimple back there.' I could tell the students were trying hard not to laugh."
SUSAN FRIEDMAN, CORAL SPRINGS, FLORIDA

A week after my surgery, our closest friends, Whit and Nancy Peyton, had John, me and the kids over for dinner. I was still wallowing in self-pity and throughout the evening, each of us took a turn at tears of despair and fear of the unknown. Suddenly Whitney turned to me and pronounced, "Chris, you *have* to find something to focus on besides your cancer."

Focus . . . focus? All I could think about was the drain dangling from my shirt and the pain I felt from the recent operation.

"I don't care if that focus becomes seeing your kids graduate from high school. You have to find something to concentrate on!" Graduate from high school? I took it for granted that I would not only see my boys graduate from high school, but college, marriage and babies no less. I wanted to be a grandmother, for Pete's sake! Of course at that moment, it was all about me: I couldn't imagine a time when I would spend more than a minute before the word *cancer* would float across my mind.

Four weeks after my surgery, I awoke in the middle of the night with a vision: cartoons. As many as fifty cancer-related cartoons started popping up in my head. I quietly worked my way downstairs in the darkness, careful not to wake my dog, Sneakers, who would eagerly eat breakfast at 3:00 A.M. if it were served to him.

I madly sketched away, and not being an artist, tried to capture the small glimpses of humor that had surfaced in the past several weeks without recognition.

"Mom, more flowers for your breast!"; "Cigarette? No thanks . . . I already have cancer"; "Mom, I shared your cancer with my class during show-and-tell!"; "Your hair looks fabulous. New hairdresser?"; "Mom, *another* pan of lasagna!"

I crept back upstairs and pulled the covers under my chin. "WHAT WAS THAT?!" I had entered the Twilight Zone, found my focus, and began my journey to seek the humor that would propel me toward recovery . . .

Schick It To Me

"*Driving to the hospital for a breast biopsy, I realized I had not shaved my legs. I told my husband that I hated to go to a doctor with hairy legs. His reply: 'If they're that far off target, you will have more important things to worry about than hair.'*"
RITA BUSCH, LAS CRUCES, NEW MEXICO

"*I was diagnosed with breast cancer and was trying to make a decision whether to have a mastectomy or lumpectomy. Explaining the differences to my grown son (fifty years old at the time), he turned to me and said, 'Mom, I'd go with the mastectomy. After all, I don't need it anymore!' "*

JUANITA C. FABULA, KANSAS CITY, MISSOURI

"I always had long hair, and I thought it would be difficult losing it during chemotherapy. The first day it started falling out, I was getting ready to go for a walk. When it started falling, I thought 'Oh my, if I go outside in the wind, it's going to blow right off!'

"I'm happy to say I only remember the silly things."

LINDA FORTI, HIBBING, MINNESOTA

"I handed out Snickers bars to the anesthesiologist and the surgeon prior to my 3:00 P.M. surgery. After all, I didn't want them to have low blood sugar in the middle of my surgery! I also had a Post-it note attached to the breast that was to be removed. It showed a cow hanging halfway over a crescent moon, with the imprinted message 'nothing in life is simple.'

"I wrote on the Post-it note: 'Dear Dr. Shmidt, before you begin cutting, please thank this breast for all it's done for me. It sacrificed itself by containing the cancer and keeping it away from the rest of my body. Be grateful along with me.' "

MARGARETE BRANDENBURG, DELPHI, INDIANA

"When I went for breast cancer surgery this year, my sister-in-law told me to make sure they had the right breast. She had to have a cyst removed a few years ago, and they started to prepare her for the wrong side. On the day of my operation, I told this to the OR nurse, who was horrified. She then proceeded to tell me about a lady who came to her

operation with a Post-it note stuck to each breast. One read, 'This is the one' and the other read, 'Hands off.' "

LYNDA BUTTERS, TORONTO, ONTARIO, CANADA

"I was waiting in my radiation oncologist's office to be marked for radiation treatments. My doctor finally saw me, and after the exam, said, 'I'll go get you scheduled for your markings. Be right back.'

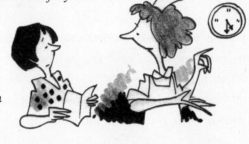

"He left the room and never returned. I waited in the room for at least another twenty minutes. Finally a nurse opened the door and exclaimed, 'What are you doing here? Everyone has gone home!' I had a good laugh! Life is wonderful!"

JOY FEELEY, PRAIRIE VILLAGE, KANSAS

Anesthesia Amnesia

When I was out,
Did I say anything really bad?
Would you tell me
If I had?

DEBORAH TRENEER PITMAN, RICHLAND, WASHINGTON

"I was told by a fellow chemo patient to be sure to wear comfortable, elastic-waist pants when going for treatments, as I would be getting *pumped full of water to assist in flushing out the chemicals, thus causing bloating and a frequent need for trips to the bathroom. Since I always like to be prepared, as well as presentable, I immediately decided to wear my jogging outfit. It was nice-looking and brightly colored. So when I sat down and promptly slid onto the floor, I decided next time cotton would be better than nylon."*

Deb Booher, langhorne, pennsylvania

Having been a business executive with nothing but stress surrounding me on a daily basis (my husband would always quip "another working emergency today, sweetheart?"), I was clueless that humor had become big business of its own. Sure, I was familiar with Norman Cousins and his groundbreaking book *Anatomy of an Illness*, but I was not prepared for the fascinating world of therapeutic humor that I would come to embrace.

It had been well documented by pioneers such as Lee Berk, M.D., and O. Carl Simonton, M.D., that laughter could provide physiological benefits such as increasing natural killer cell activity which is the body's natural fighter for viruses and tumors; increasing T-cell activity; and reducing cortison levels which tend to suppress the immune system. Dr. Edward Dunkelblau, a psychologist and past president of the Association for Applied and Therapeutic Humor describes laughter as "an aerobic experience": your breathing changes, blood flow changes, muscle tension is reduced. Stress goes down. The body responds so that the immune system is enhanced.

But besides the fact that laughter has proved to be good medicine, in its simplest terms, it feels better than crying. For a brief moment in time, the pain, humility and sadness of our disease can be turned upside down into the absurd.

"Seven years after my first surgery for cancer, lo and behold the last of November I found I had cancer again. That week they decided to put in a port because I have such bad veins. I told my dear, dear surgeon I had some questions about the port.

"Anything that requires a needle, they can do with a port. 'Give or take blood, I.V., chemo?' I asked. 'That's right,' the doctor replied. And I said, 'Well, if it does all of that, can you have sex through it?' He said, 'I give up!' Anyway; I'm hanging in there!"

ELAINE COLLIER, SELLERSBURG, INDIANA

"In November '96, I began chemo for ovarian cancer, two days after my thirty-eighth birthday. One day my husband asked me to stop by our travel agency to pick up tickets. When I walked in, the young lady sitting at the desk greeted me with 'What a great hat! You know, no one wears hats anymore. But they look so great. I think they just make an outfit. You look stunning.' And then in a whisper she asked, 'But are you having a bad hair day?' Without a pause, I said, 'No, I'm Having a No Hair Day!' When I lifted my hat up, her eyes popped out of her head! Her boss, who was standing in the doorway, turned around, went in his office and closed the door. I'm wondering if they're still having nightmares . . ."

KRIS SILVERMAN, GLENDORA, CALIFORNIA

"I have a humorous story that I wish to share with you, which proved to be my first lesson in the value of humor and lightheartedness: I came home from the hospital on March 12th, drains still in and all. The following week, on the 19th, was my thirty-sixth birthday. I was enjoying a visit from some co-workers, while unknown to only me, my roommate was on her way home with a cake. It was what we ended up referring to as 'the boob cake.' It was an actual cake with two appropriately colored breasts protruding from one end of it. It was to welcome my new breasts to the family, she said. She was nervous about bringing it home, as you might imagine. I absolutely howled with as much laughter as my incisions would allow. The experience was a hoot. We ended up saving the breasts in the freezer for after I'm finished with my reconstruction.

"I'd been feeling angry, and a bit sorry for myself. That was OK, but my birthday that year taught me that humor can be wonderfully healing, and that even though there were many things that I couldn't do physically, there were still many things left that I could do. I will always remember that birthday with a smile, and have since given laughter to many by telling the story."

KIMBERLY VEDRINSKI, WESTERVILLE, OHIO

"May I share a cartoon moment with you? Leaning over to shave my legs—head totally bald—I thought to myself, 'If I have to lose my hair, why can't it be somewhere useful?' "

LYNDA TEDESCO, VERNON, BRITISH COLUMBIA, CANADA

"I am a cancer patient and have been battling this disease for twenty-plus years. It had been in the last six years that I have had several surgeries, radiation and chemo.

"I, too, chose the positive side of this disease (if there is one . . . ha!) to try and minister to those around me. I have done things from flipping my wig in public, because in Florida it gets awfully hot, to actually going through a drive-through fast-food restaurant and taking my wig on and off each time the young person would come back to get my money and deliver my food. Poor kid . . . that was really bad of me, but my two grown girls, mom, sister and nieces got a big kick out of it."

KATHY BOWLIN, ORLANDO, FLORIDA

"The problem with a pity party? Only one person shows up and they don't serve refreshments. Keep us laughing!"

VERA TERRY, CRAWFORDSVILLE, INDIANA

"One member of our breast cancer group, Barb, had a suspicious ache in her back. We were all concerned and anxiously awaited the results of

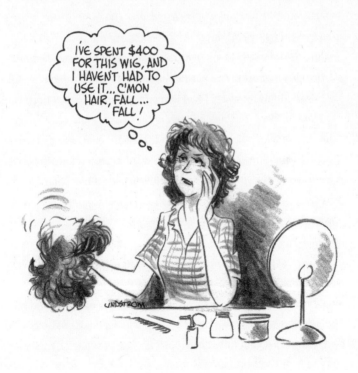

her bone scan and MRI. At the meeting following her tests, Barb cheerfully announced that she had a bulging disk, osteoporosis, and arthritis in her back, but no cancer. We all agreed that only a cancer survivor would consider those results to be good news."

JAN SLOAN, RENO, NEVADA

"Being follicily impaired at the beginning of my chemo and radiation, the loss was not a great one. But, I haven't had to shave in over two months and what has grown makes me look like a bald Colonel Sanders."

ROBERT H. MUELLER, MONTPELIER, VIRGINIA

"I was diagnosed with breast cancer in November '98 after a doctor found a golf ball–size lump in my left breast. The surgery itself wasn't so bad, but the surgically attached 'grenades' were a 'pain.' Let me explain. Sewed neatly to my right side and armpit were two separate plastic tubes that led to two plastic bottles used to collect gunk the color of Hawaiian Punch, which I will never drink again. Several times each day I had to 'bleed' the lines and record the quantity and color of the gunk. My daughter would stand outside the bathroom door and squeal 'grooooss,' making that a multi-syllable word as only young people can. It was close to Christmas and I couldn't help but wonder what Martha Stewart would make of the 'grenades': add a few sequins, some fresh greenery, candles and a pinch of marzipan and you've got a centerpiece that squirts.

"I was not to escape hospital incarceration until two criteria were met: I had to learn how to empty and clean the 'grenades.' Task number two was to listen to the wonderful Cancer Society volunteer. She opened whole new worlds for me. She'd had a double mastectomy three years before and talked about picking her prostheses. Quickly scanning her chest, she stated she had on her weekend breasts; evidently these were more understated and casual, perhaps made of flannel or denim. And then she quickly added, she also had Party Breasts. I could only imagine Dolly Parton knockers bursting forth from a sequined party dress. These breasts would glisten, these breasts would shine, these breasts would make Barbie's Ken weak with desire. She then gave me my first prosthesis (it's a good thing my mother was dead or it might have been bronzed), something I could wear home from the hospital, as if I cared. I was worried about finding a home for the two 'grenades' bulging from my sweatshirt. The prosthesis was tastefully hidden in a brown fabric bag along with numerous pamphlets from the Cancer Society. She started to giggle when I opened the bag because she had obviously misjudged my size. This breast, when alive, could have fed an entire African village.

"I could hardly wait to get home to my dog, cats and kid. My dog nearly wiggled himself to death when he saw me. After a brief greeting, the dog began to rummage through my hospital gear including the discreet brown bag. Without hesitation, he rooted around and came up with, you guessed it, the Mongo Breast! He ran around, mouth stuffed with fiberfill, shaking it furiously, making sure it was dead. If I could have snapped a picture of 'Dog with Breast,' I could have captured a real Kodak Moment, perhaps just the photo for my Christmas cards. The prosthesis eventually fell flat and was thrown away, much to the dog's dismay.

"My huge, long-haired male cat saw the 'grenade' dangling from my side, and assumed I'd been in the hospital for a permanent cat toy transplant. I felt pretty darned frisky and went out for pizza with the 'grenade' in full view. If anyone stared at the juice bottle at my side, I tried to pass it off as a colorful pager.

"All in all, I've been blessed with competent and humane medical

staff and supportive family and friends. And I
never have to be bothered with wearing a bra.
Furthermore, I can
run without
bouncing, bend
over without
anyone trying to
look down my
blouse, and swing a golf club
unencumbered. My breasts will never sag and
those tasteless jokes and cards about gravity and its effects will never
apply to me. So eat your hearts out, Baywatch babes. No-Sag Barbie is
ready to boogie."

BARBARA GRENGS, ST. PAUL, MINNESOTA

"A few weeks after I started chemotherapy for non-Hodgkin's lymphoma
and the very day I lost my hair, my husband, Gary, and I agreed to go
to our health club and work out as planned. I rummaged through a box
of scarves sent to me by a host of well-wishers and fashioned a turban
from one sent to me by my sister Linda. It was electric blue, vibrating
with psychedelic fish. I looked like the cover of a Who album.

"Halfway through my twenty minutes on the treadmill, I took off
the bandanna. Too hot. I finished my walk and went to the weights. A
woman stared at me from a stationary bike. Sweat chilled on top of my
head as the air conditioner kicked on.

"Downstairs, the locker room clattered with laughter and
conversation. There was brushing, blow-drying, styling, and spritzing
all around me, but a pained silence settled when I came to the mirror.
'Word to the wise,' I said ominously. 'Stay away from home perms.'

"They dragged their eyes away, mental wheels spinning. As I settled a
straw panama on my naked head, someone started laughing behind us.

It was the stationary bike woman. She came around the bank of lockers as I stuffed sweaty Spandex into my duffel. 'How long have you been in chemo?' she asked.

" *'Is it that obvious?'*

" *'Dang. There goes my lawsuit against Dippity-Doo.' "*

JONI RODGERS, SPRING, TEXAS

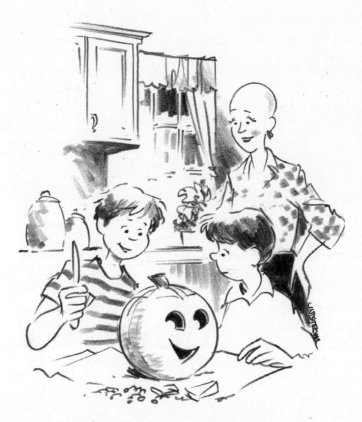

"HEY! YOU'RE RIGHT, TIM... IT DOES LOOK LIKE MOM."

CHAPTER III

Hair Loss, Doctors, Lack of Appetite? Let The Fun Begin!

A person with a sense of humor doesn't make jokes out of life, they merely recognize the ones that are there.

—AUTHOR UNKNOWN

"*Last week I was in my oncologist's office waiting room. There were two elderly gentlemen waiting to sign in at the desk where the receptionist sits behind a glass window. Before the first man could sign in, the receptionist (who is rather abrupt) says, 'Which doctor?' (asking which doctor he would be seeing that day since there are multiple doctors in their practice). The first little man's response was . . . 'Witch doctor?!!' It was so funny that the little man behind him with a hat on started laughing. I was all the way across the room and started laughing when I heard it. My husband wanted to know what I was laughing at. I told him and he started laughing. No one else in the whole waiting room knew what we were laughing at except us and the little old men. It may not be as funny to you as it was to us, but my hubby and I laughed about it all morning."*

KELLY SMITH, N. RICHLAND HILLS, TEXAS

It's a strange phenomenon what happens to people when they hear that a friend or loved one has cancer. Most people don't know what to say. They don't want to say the wrong thing, so they often end up saying nothing. A cycle of avoidance and denial only deepens the loneliness and isolation the cancer patient feels.

I found humor to be a great connector of people. After my mother's situation, I did not want to face this disease alone. I quickly found that if I could use humor to put people at ease and allow them to feel more comfortable with my diagnosis that they interpreted my humor as "having a positive attitude" and low and behold—they wanted to surround me with support.

The timing of using humor is different for every person. There does come a time for most cancer patients, however, when they realize that they cannot change their situation so they might as well make the most of it. Friends and family, often more upset than the patient at this point, certainly cannot imagine that humor might be appropriate. It is at this point in time that cancer can often bring out the very best in people . . .

I befriended a gentleman named Bill who was going through chemotherapy at the same time as me. "Captains of Chrome," we used to call ourselves as we checked our reflections in each other's shiny, bald heads.

One day, Bill came rushing up to me, all excited as if he would burst. "Christine, do you notice anything different about me?" he implored. He seemed so determined, I took my time and looked him up and down, and round and round. I shook my head in confusion. "I'm sorry, Bill. I really don't notice anything different."

"I parted my hair on the other side!"

Then there was the day I was going in for my daily radiation therapy, and an elderly gentleman was shuffling out. As we passed each other, I realized that his zipper was down and decided to offer him a courtesy.

"Excuse me, sir," I began, "I just thought I'd let you know, your fly is open."

He looked down . . . he looked up at me and said, "Honey, what can't get up, can't get out!" I figured if *he* could laugh at his situation, so could I!

I soon found I was not alone in my search for humor and discovered by viewing the humbling and humiliating things that were going on in my life in an offbeat and whimsical perspective, the unbearable became bearable . . .

"I learned that I couldn't rely on my memory, which is a side effect of chemo. During a conversation, I would ask many times if I was repeating myself because I couldn't remember if I had said my thought

out loud. I never got lost or couldn't find my way home, thank goodness. But one night, as I put dinner in the oven, I had to re-open the oven to see what I was cooking for dinner. I was very relieved to find chicken, and not the kitchen sponge."

KRIS SILVERMAN, GLENDORA, CALIFORNIA

"During one of my sister Toni's inpatient stays for treatment of non-Hodgkin's lymphoma, we learned that even the best medical treatment couldn't prevent the highballs of drugs from causing temporary deafness. We had to scream to include her in conversation. Needless to say, we quit conversing. It was a very quiet, depressing day in the hospital. Until Amy showed up.

"Amy is my mom's best friend. A laugh a minute when she's trying. Even when she's not.

"Mom and Amy decided they'd head downstairs, which was the covert language for 'I need a smoke.' Amy jumped up from her chair and followed Mom out of the room. Within seconds, the emergency staff descended upon us. They raced into the room with life resuscitating equipment. They found Toni, her husband, Jeff, and me staring at them in alarm. As we tried to figure out what happened, more staff piled in behind. All the while Toni was screaming, 'What's going on?' She couldn't hear a darn thing. Apparently, when Amy jumped up from her chair, it slid backward, rocking against the emergency call button.

" 'What?' Amy wanted to know after they returned. Just seeing her sent us into convulsions of laughter."

DAWN CHICILO, NORTH OAKS, MINNESOTA

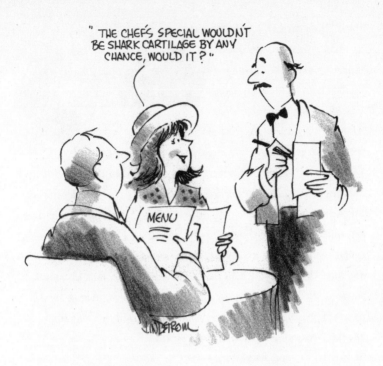

"Here's a true story for you: A patient came into radiation therapy, walked up to the front desk and said, 'I'm ready for my autopsy, I mean biopsy!' Keep laughing!"
VICKIE HILLIARD, NORTHWEST ARKANSAS RADIATION THERAPY INSTITUTE
SPRINGDALE, ARKANSAS

"Cancer is a challenge, and humor is key. I had my own 'no hair day' when I realized that upon arriving at my weekend house I had 'left my hair in the city.' My eight-year-old son and I had a good laugh with that."
PEGGY GRIEVE, NEW YORK, NEW YORK

"Wednesday, I arrived for jury duty. Harris County has a one-trial, one-day jury policy with very few exceptions. Since it was my 'off week' (from chemo), I had to show up. After spending several hours of 'hurry up and wait,' I was finally herded into a courtroom with thirty-six other poor souls. After the obligatory speeches from the attorneys, the judge asked if there was anyone among the panel who could not sit and judge this case fairly. My hand shot up without hesitation. The judge then called me to the bench where he sternly asked me why I could not sit on this jury. Did I have some preconceived prejudices against the plaintiff or the defendant? I said, 'No, sir, I am a cancer patient who is undergoing chemo and am liable to throw up at any time.' Well, the judge sat there and looked at me, then his mouth started to twitch, and he started laughing. 'That's got to be the best reason for getting out of jury duty that I have heard in a long time,' he said. Needless to say, I did not get picked."

ELIZABETH INGRAM, SPRING, TEXAS

"When my University of Florida football team (the Gators) went to the Sugar Bowl the year I was going through my treatments, I put Gator decals on my head and 'flashed' people. Their reactions were priceless!

"People sometimes say that after being diagnosed with cancer they feel like they are starting life anew. Well, that's me for sure. I now have the physique of a big, elongated, bald-headed baby. And I have the same potential a baby has, to grow in spirit and wisdom and see life with fresh eyes."

JEANNE PHILMAN, BELL, FLORIDA

"When I arrived at St. John in the room where they have the big circular Polaroid, the technician asked if I had done this before. I told her that this was number thirteen and if she wanted to take a coffee break, I could handle it by myself. She thought that was a good idea. However, after we talked it over we decided it might be too difficult for me to jump off the sliding table, run into the next room, pull the switch, run and jump back on the table in time for the ride through the big ring, and all this with my pants down around my knees. It did conjure up a heck of an active picture in my mind though."

EDWARD J. BECKWELL, ST. CLAIR SHORES, MICHIGAN

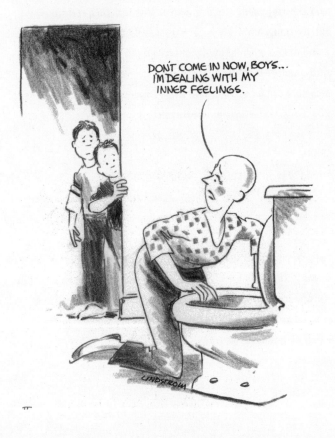

"When I was undergoing chemotherapy for colon cancer, I had terrible problems with nausea. After the first anti-nausea medication failed, I contacted my oncologist who called in an order for Compazine. Since I felt too ill to leave the house, a family member went to pick up the medication. Before taking the pills, I read the instructions, which stated, 'Put the pill in the refrigerator for 15 minutes to make sure the pill is sturdy enough.'

"I did find the instructions very puzzling. Just before I swallowed the pill, I asked my wife about the instructions and she said to me, 'Oh my gosh, didn't you know that pill is a suppository?'

"A few minutes after I inserted the pill, the phone rang. It was a very cheerful phone solicitor who asked me to do a consumer satisfaction survey. My mind was still a bit 'spaced' from the chemo, so I said to her, 'I can't now, I have a cold pill in my . . . a—' Just before I said exactly where the pill was, my wife grabbed the phone and told the person to call later. Since that time, I was told never to answer the phone right after a chemo treatment!"

EDWARD LEIGH, M.A., CLEVELAND, OHIO

"Today I went to the Department of Motor Vehicles to get my driver's license renewed. When filling out the forms, the clerk asked me if I wanted to be an organ/tissue donor. I said I would. 'Partial or Total?' 'Total.' Then I seriously began thinking, 'Maybe I should tell her I've only got one breast now—so it's Partial instead of Total.' I had this sort of Chicago Hope–like scene in my mind of a surgeon yelling 'Where's that breast transplant? We need it stat!' Then I almost cracked up laughing when I realized even my poor lonely breast wouldn't be able to be utilized!"

MARGARETE BRANDENBURG, DELPHI, INDIANA

"Nineteen years ago I underwent a sigmoid colostomy. At first, I ate at the same time every day, and all was well. I had it down pat. Getting braver, I started not wearing my bag. One day, as I was out for lunch, there were onions in my hush puppies. What a disaster! My doctor had warned me, but I thought I knew it all. Some things we just have to learn the hard way. After all these years, I still slip up at times. I travel east, west, south and north, border to border having fun and enjoying life."

EDNA P. GRESKO, RED BAY, ALABAMA

"In 1993, I was fitted for a wig by a stylist who specialized in wigs for cancer patients. When I went to pick it up after it had received a perm and styling, the stylist said, 'I'm sorry, but we have melted your wig.' They had accidently set the temperature too high and had melted the synthetic wig. It was a plastic puddle of champagne and brown colors in the little oven they used to prepare wigs. They did find and fix another wig for me—without melting it a second time."

NORMA JEAN KUHLENSCHMIDT, SELLERSBURG, INDIANA

"When I had my first encounter with the 'Big C,' being diagnosed with acute mycloid leukemia in January of 1977, a guy having no hair wasn't as much of a fashion statement as it is today.

"It was truly amazing to go walking through the local shopping mall and 'feel' the stares of all the folks who thought surely I was there to look lobotomized and sell them flowers while wearing a sari. There were even a few times that I'd go up to them and tell them that it was a government experiment gone bad, or I'd point to my head and say 'I was experiencing inward growth' (just think about it and savor the irony!).

"Nowadays with Michael Jordan and so many others who walk

around 'shaved,' it doesn't make as much of an impact but I still get my yucks. Two and a half years ago when the leukemia hit me again, I sent one of my 'naturally follicly challenged friends' an envelope with several handfuls of my hair and a tube of super glue. The last laugh was on me!"

JIM RICHARDS, JOLIET, ILLINOIS

"Looks like you've caught me lurking around. Allow me to introduce myself: 'Chemo's the name: lurking's my game. You can call me "Chem." Right now I'm on my second tour of duty in a white female, 5'4", hazel eyes, no hair. Age and weight: classified information. As for lurking, well, that's what we chemos do. We search every nook and cranny. If we find even a trace of a cancer cell, we blast it!! By the time I finish, I'll be ranked CEPE (Cancer Eradicator, par excellent)!'"

MARSHA E. COOK, RALEIGH, NORTH CAROLINA

"The preparation for a BMT [bone marrow transplant] is unbelievable. Bone marrow sampling—a trip to hell and back. My sister Toni recognized the nurse performing this inhuman procedure. She began to refuse to go through with it, but her husband, Jeff, insisted that it wasn't the same nurse that performed the first bone marrow sampling, months earlier. Observing this exchange, after the procedure was complete, the nurse asked her about it.

"Toni told her that the nurse who did the first sampling was 'a real bitch.' Smiling, the nurse couldn't help but respond. 'That was me.'

* * *

" 'Ciao!' Toni quipped, waving her hand in a good-bye gesture from her hospital bed. Our lower jaws came unhinged. Jeff and I looked at each other in shock. 'I always wanted to do that,' she said, as Dr. Chow left the room. The tugging smiles turned to smirks, as Dr. Chow would come and go. As the door swung closed behind him, our mirthful laughter echoed in return. Poor guy."

DAWN CHICILO, NORTH OAKS, MINNESOTA

Top 10 Reasons Why Losing Your Hair to Chemotherapy Is So Great

10. You can go weeks without having to shave your legs.

9. You remember what it is like to have a really good cry when your hair first falls out.

8. You can wash your face without worrying about your hair getting wet.

7. With an instant hairdo, getting ready takes a fraction of the time it used to take.

6. You can spend quality time wondering why you wore wigs in the '70s when you didn't have to.

5. You can spend your spare time wondering what your hair will look like when it grows back or if it *will* grow back.

4. You live life on the edge, wondering if your wig will flip off when you're out in public.

3. Wearing a wig includes you in an elite group: George Washington and Benjamin Franklin wore wigs, too!

2. You find that you and Dolly Parton now have even one *more* thing in common.

1. You can tell who your real friends are. They say, "That's a wig?!" and look sincerely shocked.

DIANE DAILEY, GREAT FALLS, MONTANA

Even More Benefits of Having Cancer

You don't have to do jury duty.
After the flowers die, you have plenty of baskets to fill for thank-you gifts.
You now have a nice scarf collection.
Eyebrow makeup technique is perfected.
It's okay to stay in your jammies all day.
Your vocabulary grows considerably.
You have the perfect excuse for saying "No thank you" to any food.
You have an excuse for getting The Movie Channel.
You save money on perms, haircuts, shampoo and dye jobs.
The arrival of the mail takes on new meaning.
It's easy to try a new hairstyle.
You don't have to feel guilty about gaining weight.
You can skip going to the gym for a while.
It's okay to have a "lawn guy."
No need to apologize for taking an expensive vacation.
Doctors are no longer intimidating.

Insurance companies are no longer intimidating.

You find out who your true friends are.

When it's all over, you have an excuse to plan a party.

Somebody else can do energy-consuming tasks for a while.

You can catch up on your reading.

Lots of projects on the "sometime in the future" list suddenly get done.

You can get a temporary "Handicapped" parking permit.

DEB BOOHER, LANGHORNE, PENNSYLVANIA

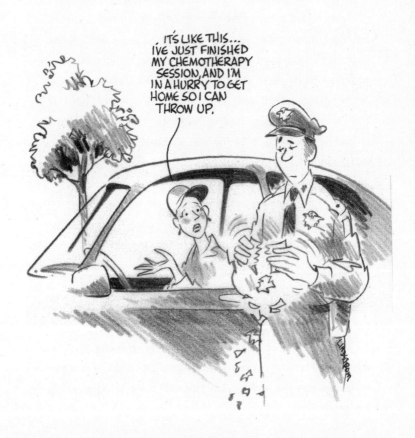

I've spoken with thousands of cancer patients who may have forgotten the sickness, baldness and fatigue, but the one thing they will always remember is that funny story or situation that made them laugh. Even if cancer patients can't fathom the association between humor and the disease, I challenge them to close their eyes and think about the number one thing that makes them laugh.

Animals, children, visual stimulation, tickling, jokes, even awkward situations can bring tears of joy instead of pools of sadness. Speaking of awkward situations, I had many as I progressed through my treatment process. Here now, a few of my favorites . . .

I grew up in a family where my father was a physician and my sister a nurse. Realizing that while I loved them both dearly and that they both had many wonderful, caring, compassionate qualities that made them experts in their fields, neither was known for being the "life of the party" or the "clinic comedian." Therefore, when I was diagnosed with cancer, the last place I expected to find humor in my situation was within the confines of the hospital and oncology clinic, which were about to become my "home away from home." But it was the words of a physician who truly brought me to my knees.

One day, months into my chemotherapy, I was trudging in for day twenty-three of radiation treatments (the "sandwich effect," I believe it is referred to), and a physician stopped me in the hall.

"Christine," he gushed, "I've heard wonderful things about you!"

"Oh, really?" I responded, immediately cheering up at what I anticipated he was about to say. After all, it could be any number of things: my job, my terrific kids, the book I was working on, my personality . . .

"Yes," he said, grabbing my arm and staring at it intently. "They say you have great veins!"

> *Blessed is he who has learned how to laugh at himself,*
> *for he shall never cease to be entertained.*
> —JOHN BOWELL

I mentioned that one of the things that often makes us laugh are awkward situations. Have you ever started laughing at something and said to yourself, "This is so inappropriate! I wish I could stop laughing!"

Like many people who have gone through chemotherapy, I lost all of my hair and I was bald as a cue ball. I always had enjoyed wearing hats, so when my hair deserted me, I ordered several special hats with the hair already attached. It was easy, and I never had to worry about how my hair looked.

I have always been a big golf fan. In fact, I have been to twenty-three straight U.S. Opens. At one point during my cancer treatments, my husband, John, and I decided to get away from the cold Minnesota winter and took a trip to Scottsdale, Arizona. There was a Senior PGA Tour event called The Tradition being played, and that seemed like just the ticket to lift my spirits.

The first day of the tournament brought out a huge gallery. It was a beautiful day, and I was in heaven. I was standing just off the third tee, behind the fairway ropes, watching my three favorite golfers in the world approach the tee box: Jack Nicklaus, Raymond Floyd and Tom Weiskopf.

Just as they arrived at the tee, the unimaginable happened. A huge gust of wind came up from out of nowhere and blew my hat and hair right off my head and into the middle of the fairway! The thousands of spectators lining the fairway fell into an awkward silence, all eyes on me. Even my golf idols were watching me, as my hair was in their flight path. I was mortified! Embarrassed as I was, I knew I couldn't just stand there. Someone had to do something to get things moving again.

So I took a deep breath, went under the ropes and out into the middle of the fairway. I grabbed my hat and hair, nestled them back on my head as best I could. Then I turned to the golfers and loudly announced, "Gentlemen, the wind is blowing from left to right." They say the laughter could be heard all the way to the nineteenth hole.

Humor surrounds us, and it is simply our ability to look at life with an offbeat and whimsical perspective that gets us through life's adversities.

CHAPTER IV

It's a Family Affair

*Let the surgeon take care to regulate the whole regimen
of the patient's life for joy and happiness,
allowing his relatives to cheer him.*
—HENRI DE MONDEVILLE, PHYSICIAN AND
SURGEON IN THE MIDDLE AGES

"While in Colorado visiting our daughter and family, our young
granddaughter, Samantha, came into the room where I was in the
process of dressing, and I as yet had nothing on above the waist. With
wide eyes, she exclaimed, 'Grandma, I didn't know you could take
your boob off!' Putting her concerns to rest and wanting her to
understand what had happened, I explained a
bit about breast cancer, showed her my
prosthesis and made a point of telling her
how thankful we can be for today's medical
know-how. Later in the evening while
overseeing bedtime preparations in the
bathroom, it was teethbrushing time for the

younger brother, Brian. He looked up at me—pointing to my teeth—

and asked, 'Grandma, what is that?' I then had to explain and show

what a 'dental partial appliance' is. He ran to the door and exclaimed,

'Come here quick, Sam, she can take her teeth off, too!' "

DOTTIE BAGSHAW, MESA, ARIZONA

It has been said that there is nothing like adversity or misfortune to teach us all how truly blessed we are. Never has that adage proved more true than to feel the love and support I received from my beloved family.

Cancer does not just affect the patient. It permeates the home environment and reaches across state lines to pull every living relative into its path. Whatever the mix of families today, be they blended or not, everyone's life in that family will be turned upside down.

It was through the love and support I received from my family that I started to realize that cancer could actually be a gift. For cancer reunited my family, from scattered places around the globe and confirmed that we would be there for each other, regardless of what was going on in each of our lives.

All of my brothers and sisters came to join me at Thanksgiving during the month I would finish my treatments. It was the first time we had all been together since my father's funeral five years prior. As we sat around the fireplace we shared our quiet pleasures and gentle joys of family ties, recalling memories that tickle your face with a smile.

★   ★   ★

Every year since my boys were little, it has been a family tradition for John and me to take them to a marvelous resort in the north woods of Minnesota appropriately named Grand View Lodge because of its spectacular perch overlooking majestic Gull Lake. It is a short three-night, four-day visit, but just long enough for us to get away from the city, relax and spend some quality time together.

We go on the same weekend, stay in the same cabin, and do almost the same things every year in an effort to establish a sense of tradition that we hope our boys will carry on for many years to come. One of our days is spent hiring a fishing guide and fishing to our heart's content (or the legal limit—whichever comes first).

The year I was going through my treatments for cancer, I was particularly looking forward to our trip as I had already been through six months of chemotherapy and thirty-three days of radiation. I knew that Grand View would be just the thing to get my mind off my situation and help me focus on positive memories of days gone by as well as dreams of future years on the lake together with my family.

On the day of our fishing excursion, the alarm went off at 5:30 A.M. so we could eat a hearty breakfast, get dressed and be on the dock by 6 A.M. It was a cloudy, overcast day—perfect for fishing. Our regular guide, Mark, showed up on time, and we took off for a day of delight.

"Mom," my youngest son, Brooks, who was eight at the time, chipped in, "are we having our annual contests?"

"You mean First Fish, Biggest Fish, and Most Fish?" asked Tim, eleven years old and already an experienced fisherman. "Ha, just watch! I'll win them all this year!" Let the competition begin . . .

We found our first fishing hole and with Mark's help, all hooks were baited and lines were dropped. An hour went by without a nibble when Mark offered to move us to another part of the lake.

Eagerly, we all dropped our lines in the quiet still of the morning, only a few signs of life starting to surface on the shore as cabin owners and guests started waking with the rising sun. Again, time sped quickly by and still not a bite. Hours passed as we would fish for a while, move to a new location and try our luck again. You could see the disappointment on the boys' faces as the day turned into afternoon and nary a fish was to be seen.

Our guide apologized up and down for our bad fortune and suggested we call it a day. Each of the boys asked if they could throw out one last cast, and we agreed as I started putting away the remnants of lunch and picking up the boat.

Suddenly, Brooks screamed with delight. "I have hooked a big one!" We all eagerly watched and waited as he struggled to pull what appeared to be a keeper through the water. He pulled and reeled, all eyes upon him when what should appear on the end of the line but the wig from the top of my head!

I gasped and reached to feel my baldness when the boys and the men burst into laughter. I could not help but laugh along with them as Brooks proudly removed my hair from his hook and announced, "First fish, biggest fish, most fish—a clean sweep!"

We laughed all the way on the ride back to Grand View, the day's disappointments far from our thoughts. Eight years have passed, and we have continued our annual trips to Grand View Lodge. Every year on several occasions throughout the weekend, someone will bring up that story, and we all laugh at the wonderful memory and the big one that almost got away . . .

* * *

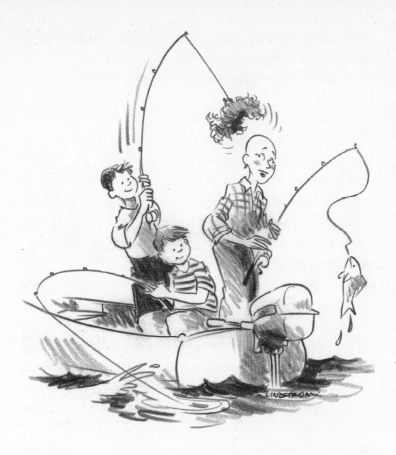

Having family members, whether they are aging parents, aunts and uncles, delightful grandparents, brothers and sisters, or even children of our own is a privilege we all have right at our fingertips.

"My four-year-old grandson, Joshua, stayed overnight one time during my chemo. He had never seen me without my scarf or a wig. I thought I better prepare him in case he woke during the night and came into our bedroom. I told Joshua I had something funny to show him. I removed my scarf and revealed my bald head. With a funny look on his face, he asked me what happened. Rather than have him fear the loss of his

hair next time he got sick, I told him I got a haircut. He replied, 'And they didn't listen, did they Grannie?!' "

MARY HARTNER, ST. MICHAEL, MINNESOTA

"Before losing my hair, I took a walk in the park with my six-year-old Maria. 'Mom,' she said, 'I saw a baby with no hair today, and you're gonna be really ugly!' Later, when my hair started falling out, I overheard her telling her friends, 'I'm selling tickets to see my mom's bald head!' "

SANDY DRESCHER-LEHMAN, RICHMOND, VIRGINIA

"I was diagnosed with colon cancer in December of '97. I was mortified at the thought of having radiation and having to 'drop my drawers' every day for six weeks. So, my husband (talented artist that he is), started drawing on my bottom. The techs loved it, and even started making requests! The last laugh was on me . . . literally!"

DEB BAUSERMAN, ROCHESTER, NEW YORK

"Like many others, I thank you for recognizing the importance of humor as we wage our wars on cancer. I was diagnosed with breast cancer on my husband's birthday in November 1998. A week later I had a mastectomy and three weeks after that I began chemotherapy. As soon as the decision was made to take my breast, the doctors told us about reconstructive surgery and the different options available. My husband voiced his opinion early on. He wanted an implant. Not just any implant. He wanted a musical one. When I asked him what the melody

should be, his first thought was 'When
The Saints Come Marching In.'
He revised that—upon a friend's
suggestion—'The Way We Were.'
We're auditioning show tunes now, but
you'll be glad to know I drew the line at
the 'Clapper' switch. There is no way I am
going to have someone walk into the
room, clap their hands and have my breast
erupt in song! I have standards!

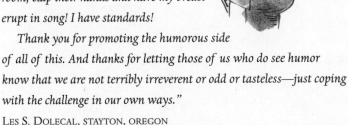

    Thank you for promoting the humorous side
of all of this. And thanks for letting those of us who do see humor
know that we are not terribly irreverent or odd or tasteless—just coping
with the challenge in our own ways."

LES S. DOLECAL, STAYTON, OREGON

"The other night my husband and I were sitting rather near each other
on the davenport when my head rubbed up next to his face. He jumps
back and says, 'Stubble, stubble.' Funny how women have put up with
whisker burns for years, and now I have a little 'after five shadow' (I
think that's what men call it), and he yells!"

JANET FLICK, WILLMAR, MINNESOTA

"As a nearly five-year survivor (September '97) of colon cancer, I
remember this: As I approached the end of a year of weekly
chemotherapy, I said to my husband, who was engrossed in ESPN,
'When I finish the chemo treatments, I'd like to go somewhere special
to celebrate.' Absentmindedly, without taking his eyes off the TV
screen, he nodded, 'Yeah, okay.' 'Like New York City,' I went on.
Instantly, he snapped to attention. His head spun around as he gasped,

New York? I thought you meant out to eat!' As it turned out, I went to Europe to celebrate instead. With his blessing, I might add.

"Thank you for all of your efforts to put an end to cancer once and for all."

CAROL S. HARTMAN, WINDOM, MINNESOTA

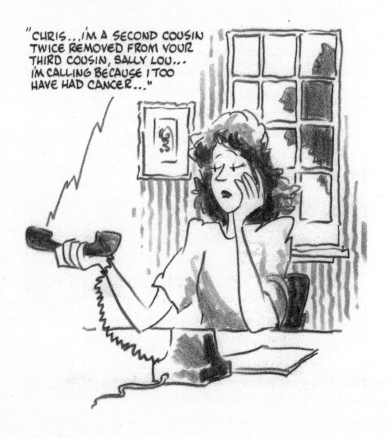

"My days following my double mastectomy and reconstructive surgery were spent wrapping, bandaging, examining, massaging, pushing up and pulling down my 'new' breasts. I was never unaware of my chest as I learned how it felt to be encased twenty-four hours a day in either a *surgical bra (more like a straitjacket!) or in an Ace bandage wrapped tight enough to prevent breathing deeply. Added to that was the occasional feeling that I was carrying around two of the state's prize-winning watermelons on my torso! My patient husband became so tired of seeing me holding, rubbing and pushing myself that he decided he had earned the privilege of grabbing his crotch every time I touched my chest! We made quite a startling pair, and of course, social invitations became nonexistent!"*

JEAN R. LOVING, RALEIGH, NORTH CAROLINA

"I had a double mastectomy two years ago. Reconstruction was done one year later and now I was deciding on where to place the nipples. One day after my husband and I had been to the plastic surgeon, who had told me to practice with round Band-Aids to visualize where I wanted the nipples to be, we were in our room trying the Band-Aids out. I would say, 'No, I think here,' he would say, 'Maybe a little more this way,' etc. Finally I hear my twenty-one-year old daughter from downstairs call out, 'What are you two doing up there?' I said, 'We are deciding where my nipples should be. Why don't you come up and give your opinion?' She did and my husband slowly slipped out of the room and let the women make the decision."

SUSAN BUSHARD, BLOOMINGTON, MINNESOTA

"How can I have anything but a wonderful day with humor in my heart? One of the funniest experiences I had during chemo was overhearing my son on the phone as I

fiddled in the kitchen. He commented to his friend, 'It's always interesting to watch Mom come home. You never know what body parts

will start coming off when she walks through the door.' Since it was
hot, I was quick to remove my wig and prosthesis . . . both rather
warm, uncomfortable items at the end of a work day!"
GRACE VERMEER, PELLA, IOWA

"I had breast cancer in 1992, at the age of forty, a single mom with a
son who was only three years old. I took my son, Quinn, with me to
radiation not because of a lack of child care, but because I wanted to
spend every second with him since I discovered I had breast cancer. The
daily hour drive, one way, to the treatment center was much more
bearable having him along, singing me songs and asking a zillion
questions as we drove through the Redwoods and past the Pacific
Ocean. At the time we lived on the beautiful north coast of California,
above Eureka.

"We got to know the hospital staff quite well. The female technician
declared Quinn her boyfriend and for the six weeks we came, she
always had a little present for him, stickers or a sucker. He was the
cutest little towhead blond, with huge blue eyes and pink cheeks, and
he would stand up on a chair, peek through a little window, as Mommy
lay on a table. I had to endure several minutes of up and down,
sideways and back as he squealed with delight watching me go through
the motions as he drove the magic table that would make Mommy
better. He and the technician would both be laughing and waving
through the window as I waved back, feeling so thankful that she was
making this experience easier on both of us.

"The radiologist was a relatively young doctor and he hadn't
impressed me much. He was quite arrogant and didn't appear to be
very caring until the day before Halloween, and my son had arrived at
the hospital with his new Batman costume on. He had worn it to show
his girlfriend. I had just finished treatment and was heading out of the

radiology room looking for Quinn, who was usually waiting right by the door. I heard giggling from the hallway and was stunned as the radiologist came running by, arms extended up in the air, carrying a flying Batman, Quinn's cape flying in the wind, his eyes wild with excitement, and screaming, 'Wheeeeeeee!' The doctor looked like he was having as much fun as Quinn. He made about three runs of the hallway. Patients, nurses and fellow doctors were in stitches. He finally put Quinn down, looked up at me panting and out of breath, and said, 'Thank you, that's the most fun I've had in a long time.' He put back on his doctor's face and continued on to his business. I felt a new respect for this man. He wasn't so arrogant after all.

"Having cancer is a tough experience; however, there are so many wonderful people that help us make it through the treatments. Thank God for them."

PENNY WALKER, SAN ANDREAS, CALIFORNIA

"My breast cancer was in October of 1991 so it's going on eleven years. Both breasts were eventually removed because of the high risk of it recurring. I don't normally wear any prostheses so one of the family jokes is that it must be something important for Mom to wear her fake boobs!! One daughter got married in 1994 and my other daughter two years later, so that's two times we know that I wore them!"

BEATRICE "BEA" NEILL, ESSEX JUNCTION, VERMONT

"One summer as I was walking to the cash register in Ross's, I saw a T-shirt in a purple and white abstract design on sale, so I picked it up without even trying it on. While cutting the labels off, I saw that the design would change color with body heat. One winter morning, I decided to wear the shirt when we went out for breakfast. After ordering breakfast, I was horrified to see that the entire shirt had turned pink except for the area around my implanted silicone breast! I rubbed on that area of the shirt to make it the same color as the rest of my shirt, and my husband pointed out that wasn't a real good thing to do in public. Great shirt sale."

RITA BUSCH, LAS CRUCES, NEW MEXICO

"A week after my first chemo treatment, my husband, Karl, walked in with his head shaved—much to everyone's surprise! When my hair started to fall out a week later, I went to my beautician, who gave me a buzz cut. Karl and I came home and looked in the mirror. Instead of crying, we started laughing! We all liked Karl's bald head so much, he still shaves his head!"

MARY ANN KING, SAVANNAH, GEORGIA

"My husband and I were watching one of those newsmagazines on TV, and they had a segment about alien sightings. My husband (of thirty-one years) said it was too bad I didn't meet one of these aliens. With my bald head they would think I was one of them and immediately come in peace!"

MARTI MARTIN, MARTINEZ, CALIFORNIA

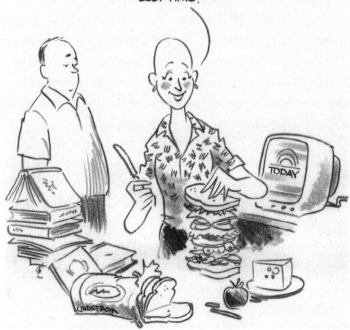

"When told I would have to have a bilateral mastectomy upon receiving a diagnosis of cancer, my husband hugged me and said, 'When we hug our hearts will be closer.' "

JEANNE PHILMAN, BELL, FLORIDA

"My white blood cell count fell several times during my six chemos. After one of the blood tests, I was told it was 1.4. The nurse made several suggestions to stay away from bacteria and viral infection. She also told me to eat only cooked vegetables. Explaining that raw vegetables had a *high bacteria count, that evening I explained to my husband that we couldn't eat any salad for a while. My eleven-year-old son came around the corner and said, 'I knew those vegetables were no good for you.'"*

KRIS SILVERMAN, GLENDORA, CALIFORNIA

"Our teenage son had a haircut appointment ten miles from our house. This is normally not a problem, but my feet were numb from chemo side effects and the only car left at home that day was the one with feather-light accelerator and brake pedals. I had a difficult time controlling the speed and my braking was less than perfect. (OK I did run that one stop sign.) I noticed a certain white-knuckled reaction to my driving performance, but had no idea about its lasting impact until the following year when my son received an 'A' for his assignment to write about 'The Scariest Experience in My Life.' He never let me read it, but I've noticed that his teachers no longer request me for field trip transportation. However, one did compliment me on enhancing my son's prayer life."

DEBORAH TRENEER PITMAN, RICHLAND, WASHINGTON

"So, there I was in the shower one morning when I found it. I yelled to my husband and he came racing into the bathroom to find out what calamity had befallen me. With an extraordinarily satisfied look upon my face, I quite proudly pointed to my armpit and told him I had a hair. It's the little things that matter."

LES S. DOLECAL, STAYTON, OREGON

"In the spring of 1994, the day after I broke the sound barrier as a Navy pilot, I was diagnosed with an almost invisible form of a cancer called amelanotic malignant melanoma on the left ear. Soon after this diagnosis, I had the jugular vein, the trapezoid muscle, the salivary gland and about 200 lymph nodes surgically removed from the left side of my face and neck. The surgeon also removed most of my left ear.

"When I finally got home from the hospital, my face and head were wrapped up tight like a mummy. Our twins, Brian and Christie, were only six years old. As soon as they saw me for the first time, they cried out 'Mummy-Daddy . . . Mummy-Daddy.'

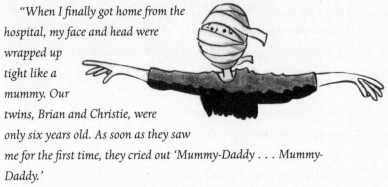

"My name became Mummy-Daddy. It would crack me up whenever I heard them say it. And even though at times it seemed almost too painful to laugh, I learned it only seemed that way, but laughter can break down any barrier, especially pain. I stayed Mummy-Daddy for quite some time.

"The doctors would not perform any plastic surgery on me until I had survived a year. Exactly one year later, a wonderfully gifted plastic surgeon reconstructed my left ear from one of my ribs that he removed, and also from a large piece of my groin.

"The operation was a complete success—except you can imagine what happens to my ear now when my wife kisses me goodnight!"

BILL GOSS, ORANGE PARK, FLORIDA

"Truth is, I'm among the luckiest of the unlucky: I've got a curable case of lymphoma and the doctors figure I have fifty years to live, which gives me time for great-grandchildren.

"At first it was thought my cat was to blame. Swollen lymph glands could be the result of cat-scratch fever, I was told, which made sense because for years we'd been pawing each other in gladiatorial sport, and if I'd been keeping score I'd say she outscratched me something like 10,000–0.

"I was ready to accept the diagnosis, swallow a pill and maybe *never even tell my mother. But Doctor Joe wanted a second opinion from the entire medical field. 'Tests,' he announced.*

"What prodding, probing, pricking procedures I didn't go through just to be told that they didn't know what I had, but that cat-scratch fever couldn't be ruled out.

"After weeks of squirming around like a porcupine in a needle stack, I cut a deal with my maker that I would never claw with the cat again if I could be guaranteed no more tests, no more needles.

"That's when they decided to operate. They pulled a node out of my groin, and I went home with a five-centimeter railroad scar to show my four-year-old girls. 'But Daddy,' one of them said, clearly shaken, 'did the nurses and the doctors see your penis?'

" 'Well, uh, yeah, I guess they did.'

" 'And did they laugh?' "

*   *   *

"My parents were not among the first to hear the news. They were traveling through Canada when the verdict came through. For two weeks I agonized over how to tell them; I practiced on others, I consulted a social worker and a psychologist.

"A few days after they returned, they came to visit us, bearing gifts and gossip and recollections of their trip. I was rolling inside, waiting for the right moment.

" 'So,' my mother said brightly, 'How have you been?'

" 'Well, actually,' I began.

"She wept. After three heart-wrenching hours of talking, crying, hugging, she admonished me. 'When I ask how you are,' she said chokingly, 'you always say, "Fine." I didn't expect you to tell me anything.'

"She'd have been happier blaming the cat. Telling my children was easier, because they didn't comprehend. I didn't look sick, so how sick could I be? We explained that I would be losing my hair—and that interested them. A couple of days later, one of them asked why I still had my hair. I assured her that it may take some time. She was aggrieved. 'It better fall out soon,' she pouted petulantly, 'because I already promised my friends.'

"Laughing about cancer has strengthened me for the fight."

SAM ORBAUM, *THE JERUSALEM POST*, JERUSALEM, ISRAEL

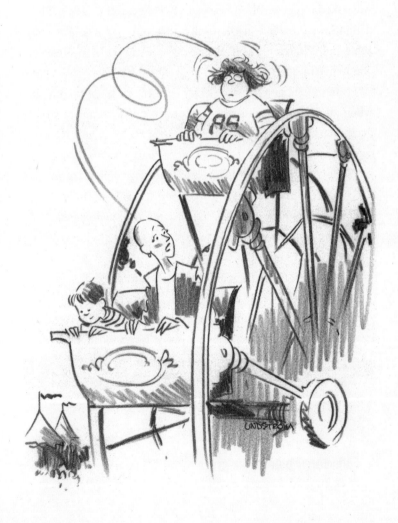

If you don't have kids in your life, I highly recommend you go out and borrow some. Start doing some volunteer work at your hospital or clinic because kids are a terrific source for humor. For one thing, they never fully understand the seriousness of the disease, which is OK. It keeps them from getting frightened.

My friend Suzie Hudson, now two years out from her diagnosis of breast cancer, remembers her daughter's reaction when she was asked to get involved in a cancer-related event. "Mom," her daughter expounded in that voice that only teenage girls can achieve, "Why would you want to go and do that? Your cancer was *so* five minutes ago!"

I can remember a Survivor's Day celebration several years ago when an elderly woman who had undergone a complete laryngectomee approached me to tell her story.

> *"I have two grandchildren," she began, her fingers pressed to her throat as her robotic voice filled the air, "David and Susan."*
> *One day Susan says to David, 'David, I can never understand Grandma's voice.'*
> *David says, 'Susan, just read her lips.'*
> *Susan replied, "David, I'm only three. I can't read!"*

We all burst into laughter, and for a while, this woman forgot her troubles and shared in the pure joy of love and laughter.

Granddaughter, Tori (3 years old)

Chemotheraphy had made me lose my hair
So on my head there was nothing there.

I wore different hats to keep my head warm.
Some of them were silly but some had charm.
Every time I'd see her, she'd check my head
To see if any of my hair had bred.
One day she said to her nanny, Sarah
(To Sarah's chagrin and probably horror),
Loudly and with much emphasis,
"Take Meme's hat off—you gotta see this!"
Now my hair is coming back in a hurry.
My head is already fuzzy and furry
And soon I'll look like her regular Meme.
The treatments and baldness will be history.
But I'll never forget her bright-eyed wonderment
That gave me precious hope and encouragement.
BETTY "MEME" CLOUGH, PLYMOUTH, MASSACHUSETTS

Let the time of trouble and worry bring your family back together. Cherish your memories, spin new stories, create a legacy for your family that will forever burn bright.

CHAPTER V

Getting By with a Little Help from My Friends

But every road is tough to me that has no friend to cheer it.
—ELIZABETH SHANE

"May I share a laugh with you, telling what happened to one friend?
Nancy was six months ahead of me in her cancer experience, and had
just had a new nipple made following breast cancer surgery. We were at
choir practice, and Nancy was anxious to
show off her nipple. A group of women went
into the church to admire the work and share
comments and chuckles. When our pastor was
sure it was safe to come in, he said, 'Did you
know the PA system was on in the chapel?' He said the only thing
heard was the laughter of friends, but we're convinced he may have
had an earful about Nancy's new nipple."
ANNIE SMITH, BROOKLIN, MAINE

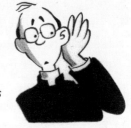

If I live to be 100 years old, I will never get over the privilege I received of seeing, while I'm still here on earth, how many people care for me and my family. It started with my closest friends, gathering 'round with a protective shield to help me make decisions, choices, find the critical care that would lead to successful recovery.

Then, one by one, day by day, I would receive a call, a card, flowers, a meal from neighbors, co-workers, acquaintances and pure strangers. I was in treatment, from surgery on New Year's Eve through chemotherapy and radiation, finishing eleven months later. Not one single day went by that I didn't hear from someone, somewhere, and that feeling of unconditional support became a feeling of empowerment for me to recover that much more quickly, strongly and fully. I didn't want to let anyone down! You can learn a lot about your friends when misfortune comes into your life. You will discover who your true friends are, and who your true friends aren't.

From the extraordinary gestures to the ordinary, I learned that the lengths that people will go to help a friend are often unexpected, highly unusual, and always humorous . . .

Among those whom I like or admire, I can find no common
denominator, but among those whom I love,
I can: all of them make me laugh.

—W. H. Auden

"I want to share a cute name that my co-worker John has come up with since I have been going through CMF chemotherapy for breast cancer for the past five months. John is a person with a great sense of humor and he, as well as my other colleagues, have helped me cope with this disease and its treatment in so many wonderful ways. His nickname: 'CHEMO-SA-BE.' I get a big chuckle out of this and wanted to share this enjoyable and funny moment with other survivors."

Nancy Roberts, Pasadena, Maryland

"Shortly following chemotherapy and on one of my earliest outings without a wig, sporting a one-inch haircut, I was searching for a pin to match a set of earrings. A friend and I were at a craft show outdoors where there were many merchants, shoppers, and folks just enjoying the weather. Lo and behold, there was the perfect pin. Unabashedly, my friend spotted another item, and in an excited voice said, 'Oh, look Deb! Here's a matching barrette!' When she realized her error, she looked at me with that stricken 'What have I done?!' face, and all I could do was burst into laughter at the absurdity of it all. Needless to say, the onlookers thought we had lost it."

Deb Booher, Langhorne, Pennsylvania

"A couple of years ago my sister's friend Barb (early 50s and married for many years) was diagnosed with vaginal cancer. Barb asked my sister to sit in with her while the doctor explained things to her. After the doctor explained the proposed surgery, radiation and chemotherapy, he assured her she would be able to return to her 'normal' sex life when it was over. Barb turned to my sister and said, 'Boy, there is no good news about this cancer!'

"Barb (who has always battled a weight problem) made her girlfriends promise that if she dropped to under 110 pounds, they would bring her to the department store to try on size six clothes—even if they had to push her in a gurney.

"Barb is doing great now, by the way."

MARNO JOHNSON, NORTH OAKS, MINNESOTA

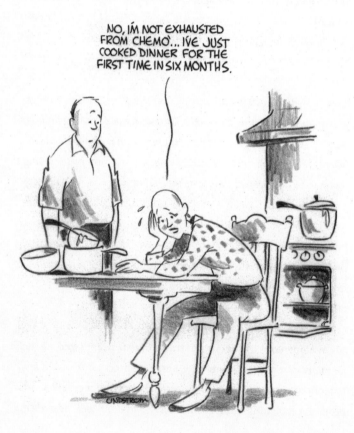

"I'm well again, baruch hashem, in'shallah, thank God and Hadassah-University Hospital both. To those who prayed for me I thank you, and let you take credit for my recovery; to those who wrote, faxed, called and patted me on the arm, you, too, get credit, for galvanizing my will and lifting my spirit. (And to all the people who didn't pray, write, fax or call: I know who you are.)

"Oh, it was wonderful that everyone had to be nice to me, forgiving me at my most cantankerous. It was a rare privilege to hear so many eulogies that one usually gets in one's life only a day too late."

SAM ORBAUM, *JERUSALEM POST*, JERUSALEM, ISRAEL

"One night at a party with friends, I must have told my story five or six times that night to different people. Even I got bored with the same story. Of course everyone thinks that if someone is sick they need to be hugged. Don't get me wrong, I'm the first one to enjoy a good hug. Now with my white blood cell count so low, all I could think of was how many germs I was hugging. The topper was a friend who asked me how I was. Put on her 'I'm so sorry for you' face. Hugged me. Then reported to me that she, too, wasn't feeling well. That she had been home ill with the flu, and that she caught it from her son, who had been out of school for two weeks. Oh great, this lady is feeling sorry for me on one hand and is Typhoid Mary on the other.

"I have some wonderful friends who took very good care of me. Some made me laugh. Some made me dinner. Some took care of my children. Some sent cards weekly. I cherish all those things. But I was the one going through chemo, so some of the things people said I just had to laugh at. Many people were curious about my hair loss, no big deal. I often went bald around the house. Every opportunity I laughed about having no hair. Many people said, 'You know, my other friend went through chemo. And her hair came in curly. Maybe yours will, too.' After hearing that over and over I came to the conclusion, that to the people who had not been through chemo, getting curly hair was a benefit. I think I'd rather have straight hair. Right now I'd rather have any hair.

"I even had a friend say, 'A friend of mine had colored her hair so long she didn't know what color it was anymore. Then when her chemo was over, her hair came in a lovely silver. She was quite surprised.' Well, I'd be surprised if my hair came in silver, too. Somehow I think that story was supposed to make me feel better. Somehow."

KRIS SILVERMAN, GLENDORA, CALIFORNIA

"I had just been elected to the U.S. Congress for my first term when I was diagnosed with breast cancer. While speaking at a Cancer Society event (six months later), I was explaining my reaction to a Reach to Recovery volunteer who visited me in the hospital after my mastectomy. She had on a fitted knit dress and looked fabulous. I couldn't believe she had had a mastectomy. She finally said to me, 'Just put your hands on my breasts and tell me which one I had removed.'

"Without missing a beat a man stood up in the back of the room and declared loudly, 'I'd do that for you anytime, Barbara.' Thanks to him, I learned to laugh rather than cry."

BARBARA VUCANOVICH, UNITED STATES CONGRESSWOMAN, RENO, NEVADA

"My story is about my nephrectomy scar that goes from my spine to my navel around the right-hand side of my body, along the bottom of the rib cage, in a big giant swoop. My wife says that it looks like I was attacked by a swordsman.

"I was changing at karate from my karate uniform into my street clothes, and a new member saw my scar and looked at me with a little bit of fear in his eyes. Before I told him the truth, I said that I had a teacher attack me with a sword in class. Then I told him, 'You should see how bad the other guy looks.'

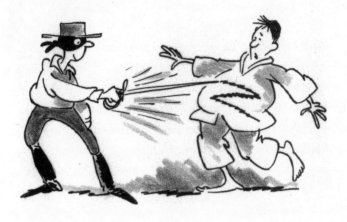

"Another time was two months after my surgery. My wife and I went to Key West and were getting ready to get out of a small boat, about twenty minutes from land for an hour of snorkeling. The water was rough, and there was no land in sight. I took off my T-shirt, and a fellow passenger looked at me in shock but wouldn't say anything. I told him 'I got attacked by a shark right here and I promised myself that wouldn't stop me from going back in the water!' Of course I told him later that it was surgery unrelated to sharks, but he waited for me to go in first before he did."

BARRY SUMMERS, NEWTOWN, PENNSYLVANIA

"After my lumpectomy, eating out with friends, we discussed my upcoming treatments, surgery, etc. We then had lunch, talking about everything that was happening to me. Just when we were getting up to

leave, one friend touched my arm and said,
'What do you use for stuffing?'

   "I immediately replied, 'Stove Top.'
We all laughed for ten minutes!"

MARILYN HILTIBRAN, URBANA, OHIO

"I had a lumpectomy on December 18, 1996, but
for eight days in late November I thought I was
going to have a mastectomy and attempted to
prepare myself for that traumatic event. During that
time, as a divorced woman wondering about the effect my new body
would have on my dating life, I had the following thoughts. Someone
should make a bumper sticker that reads, 'Real men don't need breasts.'
If I were to go out with a man who didn't know my boundaries and he
tried to fondle my left breast, which would actually be a prosthesis, I
could blow him away by offering, 'Just a moment and I'll get that out
for you; it will be easier,' or if he tried it with my right breast, I'd have
to ask him to switch to the left, and he'd wonder what difference it
made."

MELANIE PATZKOWSKI, LA MIRADA, CALIFORNIA

Then, of course, I had the friend who was using a dating service
at the time of her cancer treatments. Getting a "hot" prospect on
the line, she asked point blank, "Do you do bald?"

In Sickness and In Health

   In the beginning,
   He helped me wash my hair
   And put on my socks.

In the middle,
He helped me wash my socks
And put on my hair.

In the end,
We walked together barefoot without a care
While the wind blew softly through our hair.

DEBORAH TRENEER PITMAN, RICHLAND, WASHINGTON

The following poem summarizes so much of what we all struggle with as both cancer patients and the friends who love us. I've always felt that the most important thing a friend could do would just be to acknowledge that they've heard about what we are

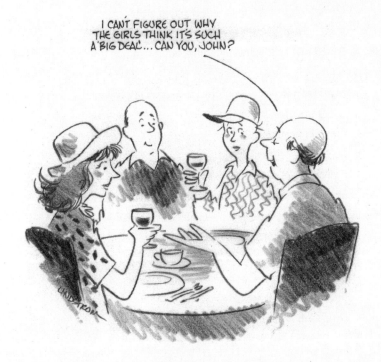

going through and we are in their prayers. It's the friends who don't say anything that cause more pain and sorrow.

Comforters

When I was diagnosed with Cancer:
My first friend came and expressed his shock by saying,
"I can't believe that you have cancer.
I always thought you were so active and healthy."
He left and I felt alienated and somehow very "different."

My second friend came and brought me information about
different treatments being used for cancer. He said,
"Whatever you do, don't take chemotherapy.
It's a poison!"
He left and I felt scared and confused.

My third friend came and tried to answer my "whys?"
with the statement "Perhaps God is disciplining you for
some sin in your life?"
He left and I felt guilty.

My fourth friend came and told me,
"If your faith is just great enough God will heal you."
He left and I felt my faith must be inadequate.

My fifth friend came and told me to remember that
"All things work together for good."
He left and I felt angry.

My sixth friend never came at all.
I felt sad and alone.

My seventh friend came and held my hand and said,
"I care, I'm here, I want to help you through this."
He left and I felt loved!

LINDA MAE RICHARDSON, WICHITA, KANSAS

CHAPTER VI

The Power of Passion and Creativity

The limitless potential which is the basis for all that any of us can and have become is brought forward by our sense of humor and laughter.

—AUTHOR UNKNOWN

"I, too, found that love, support and a healthy dose of laughter really got me through (my bout of breast cancer). My hardest time was a trip to M. D. Anderson for a second opinion. We all felt a little down and decided we must bring a 'Celebration of Life' home with us. That's when we found 'Daisey'—a 5'7½" giraffe topiary. She weighs 150 lbs. and has her own watering system. She lives in our front yard and brings smiles to all who ride the streetcar in front of our *house. We decorate her for every occasion. Daisey and I had a*

Celebration of Life Party when I finished my chemo. Isn't life

wonderful, precious and so fragile!"

VAL KEHOE, NEW ORLEANS, LOUISIANA

Cancer patients and survivors are among the most creative people on earth. Cancer can often bring out the passion in people: The creativity and growth that is so very often experienced in cancer patients is a tribute to what we've all been through and faced. Creativity is a life-affirming experience that tells the world, "I've faced adversity, but I'm not ready to give up yet!"

Our world is a better place thanks to the gifts we've been given by those whose lives have been touched by cancer: the poetry, art, stories and novels, plays, movies, photography, crafts and creations. Don't tell yourself "I can't do it." Get going *today* and create something for a friend or loved one. You'll both treasure it for the rest of your lives.

Cancer can also be the catalyst to helping us achieve our dreams. Rather than thinking, "I have cancer. Now I'll never achieve my dreams," a cancer experience can allow you the opportunity to reflect back on your life and gives you permission to make the changes that you've always wanted to make.

From the time I was a young girl, I had dreamt of becoming an author. Throughout my youth I cherished creative writing assignments, and upon entering college, even majored for a brief period in journalism.

My mother's death forced an abrupt end to my college education, and reality set in quickly as I was forced to find a "real job" in the middle of my junior year. Through perseverance, luck and timing, my career led me on a path that far surpassed my wildest expectations, and over time I rose to the level of senior executive vice president of an international marketing company.

My writing skills were left to training manuals, memos, minutes and the occasional "white paper," but whenever people would read anything I wrote ("thank-you notes" were my specialty), they would always say, "Christine, you should be a writer."

I heard the phrase so frequently that I thought long and hard about why I had never pursued my passion. The same answer always floated to the top of my list: I couldn't think of a subject that I felt I knew enough about to put a pen to paper.

Following that infamous night I had four weeks after my surgery, when I awoke in the night and started scribbling cartoons, the next day I got up, dressed, and went to both the public library and a Barnes & Noble bookstore. I strode into the bookstore first, walked up to the information counter, and announced, "I'd like to see all of your humorous books about cancer, please." The clerk behind the counter squinted his eye as he looked at me disdainfully and pronounced, "You're sick." Aha! I chuckled to myself as I pulled a notepad out of my purse, scribbling down his very words: another cartoon for my book!

I proceeded across the street to the library where I was guided to one book technically classified under "Humor and Cancer": Erma Bombeck's *I Want to Go to Boise, I Want to Grow Up, I Want to Grow Hair*. "I think I'm on to something," I thought gleefully as I pulled out of the parking lot and headed toward my daily radiation therapy.

Days, weeks, months passed by as I trudged on through my

treatments. My cartoons and "my book" became my focus as I searched for signs of humor in my predicament. The harder I looked the more I found, and my first book *Not Now . . . I'm Having a No Hair Day!* was born.

Exactly one year from the day I sat in the hospital recovering from cancer surgery, I sat in my publisher's office and signed a contract for not one, but two books about using humor as a tool to deal with a diagnosis of cancer. Both of my books, . . . *No Hair Day* and *Our Family Has Cancer, Too!* written especially for children, have won awards and received international acclaim and media attention.

I look back on the many roles I have played in my life: daughter, sister, student, wife, mother, businesswoman, entrepreneur, professional speaker, fund-raiser, friend, cancer survivor.

But the role that I hold dearest to my heart and fills me with pride is that of "author." Today is the perfect time to dream . . .

"I currently have a part-time position, which allows me the freedom to play golf as much as possible. Due to sheer determination (and a lymph node dissection on my right side in 1996!), my handicap has come down to eighteen strokes in the past two years! Luckily, no lymph node dissection was required in December on my left side, so my follow-through has not been altered!

"First things first!"

MARY WEIDENSAUL, GRANBY, MASSACHUSETTS

"In the latter 1970s while working for a Ph.D. at Caltech, I began gradually losing my visual field. Finally, five days before I was scheduled to take my final oral exam over my Ph.D. thesis, evidence was found that it was a large growing tumor from the pituitary gland

that was destroying my optic nerve. *(Well, apparently an old college buddy of mine was right after all when he suggested I needed brain surgery!) Knowing that I was about to go before five of Caltech's finest, I was reserving judgment as to which was worse: the final oral exam or the surgery!*

"I passed my final oral exam without difficulty, so the pituitary tumor became a significant 'gift' to go with my degree—one that I will never forget!"

CROCKETT LANE GRABBE, PH.D., IOWA CITY, IOWA

"I hope you find this 'uplifting.'"

Post Mastectomies

"You'd not know they were gone,
If you weren't snoopy;
One small consolation:
What's left isn't droopy!"

JOAN T. MULLER, VERO BEACH, FLORIDA

"When I entered the hospital for cancer surgery, my friends presented me with a book of limericks they had written, and we've been adding to it ever since."

To the hospital you go when you're sick
In your arms, the needles they stick
You don't get good rest
The food's not the best
Get well and get out of there quick!
(Dr. Laurie Goldsticker)

After surgery, the nurses tried to get me to have a bowel movement, but
I hadn't eaten in nearly seven days!

> *Leslie was a sweet young lass*
> *Whom the nurses did certainly harass*
> *'It takes more than soup*
> *to make someone poop*
> *We can't send you home with just gas!'*
> *(Dr. Laurie Goldsticker)*

During chemotherapy, I couldn't eat a thing and couldn't eat meat at all.

> *My mother keeps offering treats*
> *But taxol's too taxing for eats*
> *When three hours are up*
> *I'll be ready to sup*
> *On veggies and fruits but not meats.*
> *(Jeanne Marcus)*

Finally, one friend asked if there was anything off-limits.
'Hair is not a funny subject.' I lightened up toward the end.

> *I looked under the wig that I wear*
> *And I said to myself 'I declare,*
> *Much to my surprise*
> *With my very own eyes*
> *I see 1.3 inches of hair!'* "

LESLIE MARCUS AUERBACH, NORFOLK, VIRGINIA

"You may find of interest the poem I wrote and posted on my office door
when I went for breast cancer surgery after New Year's:

"*There once was a lawyer named Betsy*
Whose breast cells became a bit testy.
The surgeon gave her a whack
It landed her flat on her back—
But soon she regained her full zesty!

"*My dad's comment on breast exams: 'In high school, he used to perform*
them regularly on his dates. They were usually very grateful!' "
BETSY SEASTRUM, WASHINGTON, D.C

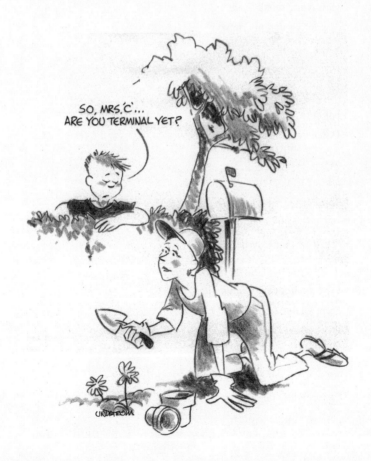

Hair Today Gone Tomorrow

When taking my treatments
There was hair in the air
It was mine and it shed
There was hair everywhere!

When I lay on my pillow
I left behind hair
Hair clung to my husband
My clothes and my chair.

I knew, but there's really
No way to prepare
For how funny you look
When you lose all your hair.

I hate to complain
And hate to sound whiny
Without hair on my scalp
My head's looking shiny.

Why do magazines now
Seem all about hair
Best cuts, perms and color
And best styles to wear?

I'm yearning for lashes
For eyebrows and hair

I'm ready and waiting
For hair everywhere!

Jeanne Philman, Bell, Florida

A Message to My Cancer

We can sir, we will sir, overcome you, vile cancer.
To stop your invasion there must be an answer.

We have radiation and chemo to slow your attack,
And medications to keep you from coming right back.

Besides doctors and nurses, hard at work behind scenes
Are researchers, technicians and their high-tech machines.

I'm thankful to them—they're all on my side
Against you—this monster from which none can hide.

For my part, I'll try hard to keep hope alive;
For a happy attitude I surely will strive.

This is aided of course by my family's love,
And many answers to prayer from the Lord up above.

It's a powerful team that you're up against—
Which, sir cancer, by now you surely have sensed.
From my body, we plan to evict you, you know,
And crush out your power—no mercy, we'll show.

Doris Kredit, Corsica, South Dakota

Bionic Woman

(geriatrically speaking)
Two new lenses in my eyes,
Prosthesis on my chest,
Bridgework brightens up my smile,
My hearing-aid's the best;
My knee replacement's working well,
My head's demurely wigged,
A pacemaker completes my gear;
I'm truly geri-rigged.

Mastectomy Musings

(with apologies to Cole Porter and others as necessary)
1) To my surgeon:
I got you under my skin!
You slashed, and came all the way in,
You excised the "crud" with some
tissue—and blood—
Now I'm flat where my breast had once been.

2) To my mirror:
But how could I think I'd stay flat
When my wound is surrounded by fat?
Now an under-arm pouch
makes me fidget and slouch—
(Has my breast been transformed into that?)

3) To myself:
Oh, stop being silly and vain!
(There's no reason at all to complain)
Just sound the "Hurrahs"
for mastectomy bras:
I've recovered my figure again!

JANET M. WEISS, MINNEAPOLIS, MINNESOTA

Life

Crisis and sorrow confront us
At times when we're least prepared.
They sap us of hope and commitment
To face our concerns and cares.

If we let all our ills defeat us,
And give in to our fears and stress,
We cease to have opportunity—
Our hope becomes less and less.

But if we reach and catch a sunbeam
That propels our spirit high,
We can learn to make connections
That give us the strength of life.

Laughter

The whispers say
"Why does she smile?"
"Why does she look so happy?"

They do not know
The chaos within her breast.
They do not know
That cancer found a place.

Surgery excises the cancer
And radiation zaps the rest.

But it is laughter that heals the spirit
And renews the will of life.
Laughter conquers the illness
And puts radiance in her face.

PEGGY STEVENS, LAKESIDE, MI

It was Doc found the lump in my breast,
Not myself, nor when mammogram pressed,
As we lay in the house.
(Yes, the doctor's my spouse.)
And for fun, I think this method's best.

Now let me allay any fears.
It was cancer, but do not shed tears.
I was sliced, I was fried,
I took poison inside,
And in June it's exactly ten years.

CAROLYN FARKAS, ELKTON, MARYLAND

It's gone, it's gone, it's no longer there!
Perhaps it lies in the trash somewhere!
It may seem perverse, this small bit of verse,
But there's long been a rumor,
As to my sense of humor.

There's just nothing to do as I lie here in bed,
And all kinds of thoughts run through my head.
Where did it go—this poor breast of mine.
This breast of mine that once was so fine.
Perhaps in a jar in chemical fizz.
I wonder where this breast of mine is!
Maybe they'll say "Oh, look it's a breast!"
Perhaps they'll be a wee bit impressed!
But I don't care if they gape and they stare.
The breast that I lost was just one of a pair.
They'll make me a new one of foam or of gel.
One that I'm certain will serve me quite well.
All women have breasts, it's part of our make-up.
And something like this gives us call to wake up.
The end of a breast is not the end of living.
We still can go on and be loving and giving.
Now's not the time for crying and moping.
But rather the time for coping and hoping!

KYRA ECKLES, RIVERSIDE, CALIFORNIA

Christine Clifford's Cancer Club

Cancer Survivor's what I am
Cheers to bring you if I can!
Courage, comfort, I understand
Creating laughter's in my hands!

Club brings smiles continuously
Contains day brightners as you'll see!
Caring and sharing with cheer I believe
Could conquer, help cure eventually!

KAY ITZIN, BROOKLYN PARK, MINNESOTA

Gory Story

The Surgical Drive-Thru is here.
First thing, you empty your purse.
And if you think that is barbaric,
Stick around: it gets even worse.

Anesthesia? Forget about that:
They tell you to "bite the bullet."
And they don't even push your gurney—
You simply hop off—and you pull it.

The appendage, of course, is removed—
Whacked off—as clean as you please.
Thank goodness this isn't Great Britain:
They might say it was MAD COW Disease.

Let your husband wait upon you
To prove he's the "salt of the Earth,"
And if you'll excuse the expression,
"Milk it" for all that it's worth.

I'll say this for them: they're efficient.
You are OUT in a couple of hours;
No need for a bedside manner—
No visitors, candy, or flowers.

One side of your bra is empty.
What the heck; just stuff it and "fudge it."
(If Bill Clinton thinks he has problems,
All he has to balance: The Budget!)
JOAN T. MULLER, VERO BEACH, FLORIDA

Still Me!

He lost a leg. "Don't fret," they said, "you're still the man we
  knew."
She lost a hand. "Poor dear," they said, "we still will stand by you."
She got MS. "We'll help," they said, "each time you need support."
His heart attack. "Hang in," they said, "we're all here for you,
  sport."

I lost my breasts. "Too bad, you're not a woman anymore."
I proved them wrong. Fought cancer—won! Now I'm better than
  before.
I know a woman's not her breasts—she's heart and mind and soul.

*And my TRUE friends and family know that I'M STILL TRULY
WHOLE!*

CATHY BARCHECK, CINCINATTI, OHIO

We may not all be poets or writers, but sometimes passion and creativity come through in the gifts people create for us as patients.

"In January of 1998, I was diagnosed with Stage IV breast cancer. My whole family listened as my doctor explained that he was going to pull out all stops, and treat the disease with vengeance. As I contemplated the path ahead of me, I decided that I would need to gather all the resources possible: my faith, family, friends and a healthy dose of fun and laughter. However, something was missing. I needed a visual representation to remind me of my many blessings as I traveled on my 'Journey of Hope.'

"How could I focus on the gifts rather than the pain of each new day? How could I invite family and friends to participate without becoming a burden on them? As I sat contemplating my dilemma, my eye caught the beautiful glass bowl given by a dear friend. We never knew exactly what it was for, so it just sat in the den collecting dust. Suddenly my mind was humming! I would collect marbles. Each morning I would put one clear marble in my bowl! It would represent my hopes for the day: sunshine, afternoon tea, a warm fire or just feeling well enough to take a stroll around the house. Each night, a colored marble placed in the bowl would represent my thanks: a visit from a dear friend, a get-well message or the healing touch of a hug.

"I could never have dreamed what an important role these little marbles would play in my healing. Family and friends immediately became involved. I received marbles from as far as Cairo, Egypt, and as

near as the young boy across the street. Many marbles arrived in pairs, clear and colored accompanied by notes of good cheer. Family and friends were invited to share in the daily ritual. They too stopped to appreciate the many small gifts that often go unnoticed in our busy lives.

"My treatment is over now but the lesson of the marbles remains close to my heart. My illness and those marbles have helped me to appreciate my many gifts. I try to live in the precious presence each day and appreciate the alrightness of what is.

"Today, when I pass through my den and see the sunlight streaming through my beautiful bowl of marbles, I stop and give thanks for the greatest gift of all, LIFE."

VAL KEHOE, NEW ORLEANS, LOUISIANA

"I was kind of upset when a niece mentioned that my sisters had planned a 'living quilt' for the project at this year's family reunion. It was too late for me to make a square. I was teaching summer school, so I arrived two days after everyone else. When I got to the reunion, the quilt was almost finished. That first night at the big family dinner, my sisters brought the quilt out and asked me to come up and look at it. Suddenly, I realized everyone was watching me. You cannot imagine how stunned I was when I began to read each square. My sister Sally got up to make the presentation. She said, 'We want you to take this home, so each night you can wrap up in the love of your family.' They had left a square open for me, and on it I wrote, 'MY success is the sum of all who love me.' "

MARY MINOR, LAFAYETTE, LOUISIANA

"Here I am—fourteen years of PMS! No, not fourteen years of Premenstrual Syndrome but fourteen years as a Postmastectomy Survivor!

"At age forty-three, after bathing and doing my breast self-exam, I discovered a lump. A mastectomy was done with the diagnosis of tubular carcinoma—no lymph node involvement. I did not have chemo or reconstruction. What I did have was five years of severe anxiety and numerous hospitalizations on a mental health unit! Some relatives thought I was 'mental' and would not recover!

"Eventually, I gained spiritual and physical strength, took charge of my life and tossed the pills and psychiatrists!

"Three times I represented my state nationally at pageants in Las Vegas and Reno, Nevada, as Ms. South Dakota United States of America, Mrs. South Dakota United States and Ms. South Dakota US of A. I was recognized on the syndicated television program Extra. On Labor Day, 1996, I placed the monetary total on the tote board at a local television station for the Jerry Lewis Stars Across America Telethon. The summer of 1997 I was chosen to appear in the July swimsuit edition of the Golden Times state publication and also was selected as a Bellissima finalist at their photo modeling agency in Santa Rosa, CA.

"I love to laugh and keep abreast (pun intended) of life!"

VAL OHRT, SIOUX FALLS, SOUTH DAKOTA

In 2000 Nobel literature laureate Gabriel Garcia Marquez said that having received his diagnosis of lymphatic cancer was an "enormous stroke of luck" that pushed him to write his memoirs. Lance Armstrong, diagnosed with Stage IV testicular cancer in 1996, turned the cancer community upside down with his victories in the world's most prestigious bicycle race, the Tour de France in 1999, 2000 and 2001 only two years after his battle with cancer. And in 1999 Dr. Jerri Nielsen treated her own diagnosis of breast cancer while working at a South Pole research station until she was rescued by the United States Air Force. Cancer does not mean that we have to crawl in a hole and give up. It can be the beginning of a new life, a creative life that propels us toward our greatest successes.

> *Don't divide your life into weeks, months or years.*
> *Rather divide your day into moments.*
> *Then live each moment as if it were one full life.*
> —AUTHOR UNKNOWN

CHAPTER VII

The Halo of Hope

*Humor is the prelude to faith and
laughter is the beginning of prayer.*
—REINHOLD NIEBUHR

"*I am still winding my way through the chemotherapy adventure and
have recently switched from some harsh chemicals to Taxol. As a result,
I will be losing my eyebrows
and eyelashes and any other
remaining hair. I started Taxol
on Ash Wednesday so I'm all set—I'm
giving up eyebrows for Lent. If only I
was Catholic!*"

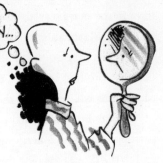

LES DOLECAL, STAYTON, OREGON

Faith and a positive attitude can go a long way toward making a cancer experience bearable. Each and every day is precious to us . . . a gift from heaven.

Cancer brings time for change, resolution, promises and commitment. As we reflect back on all the things that have taken place in our lives since we received our diagnosis, don't we all have a lot to be thankful for?

The day holds so much promise. Only months ago the headlines in the news blared, "Cancer deaths fall for the first time in decades!" Maybe this will be the day they find the cause.

The day holds so much hope. New drugs are developed every day that prolong our lives, ease the pain, suppress the disease. Maybe this will be the day they discover a guaranteed treatment.

The day holds so much passion. There are physicians, scientists, politicians and clergy who are all doing research to put an end to the disease. Maybe this will be the day they find a cure.

So make a resolution: to maintain a positive and healthy attitude each and every day, so that this time next year, we'll all be able to say, "See, we did it again! It's another year!"

This thing called cancer would I'm told,
Linger 'round if it could,
And might even become rather bold.

My job was to defend
With any resources I could.
In order that my body could mend
And fight this "invader"—as it should.

Breast and lymph nodes were removed.
My "filling stations" were located elsewhere.
My bag of healing tricks would include
Rest, treatment, nutrition, kindness, humor and facing fear.

I didn't feel any less
My persona was still whole
Having undergone this test
Better character to mold.

As a survivor let me say
Treasure the moment, sprinkle a little love
Value each day
Give thanks to Heaven above.

MARGARET JENKINS, SEAFORD, VIRGINIA

"My motto is the same as my blood type: B Positive!"
—CYNTHIA NELMS

"You project such a refreshing attitude about a serious subject—and
that's at least half the battle right there. If only that message could
reach everyone (and their families!) who have dealt with cancer, what
a difference it could make. Humor used in the same breath as the "C"
word—you bet! When you lose your ability to smile or laugh, you die a
little inside. Even God has a sense of humor—just look around you. I

guess if someone were to ask me what I once had that I no longer have and will never have again, I'd say 'cleavage' (and that's my sick humor for the day)!"

HELEN HOPE, ST. CROIX FALLS, WISCONSIN

A Better Chance

(written for Christine Clifford)
Cancer has its privileges:
I look like Captain Picard.
My husband may finally do the dishes,
He doesn't want me working too hard.

But the main privilege is
That I am still alive today.
And I can share with you
The value of life in a humorous way.

Martin Mull said,
"Life is better than death;"
Well, it could be
but don't hold your breath.

My family history says cancer could strike me.
Thank God, I heard of The Cancer Club® in advance.
I am preparing by laughing: often, loud and strong.
Now, if I do get cancer, I'll have a better chance!

STEPHEN HUNT, THE WIZARD OF HA-HAs, CEDAR RAPIDS, IOWA

A cheerful heart is good medicine,
but a downcast spirit dries up the bones.

—PROVERBS 17:22 KJV

"I have had several laughs through the last few months. They told my three-year-old grandson that my hair might come back in a different color. He called me one night and said, 'Mammy, will God let your hair come back in green?!' (His favorite color.) One Sunday in church I was playing the organ, and I had just happened to wear my wig that day. He looked up and noticed it, and hollered, 'Mammy, you got your hair back!' The preacher had to quit his sermon right there. I have just finished eight months of chemo and in August I had a bone marrow transplant. Keep smiling!"

CAROLYN WATSON, ASTORIA, ILLINOIS

"A little over twelve years ago, I received a gift. It wasn't the usual kind of gift one eagerly unwraps with anticipation. The package was quite unsightly and unsettling. Its wrappings were cancer and chemotherapy. The ribbons on the package were not the usually bright-colored decorations one expects. No, these ribbons were the dread colors of despair, frustration and suffering. Why did I receive such a repulsive 'gift'? I chose not to let this question haunt me. I concluded that everyone receives unsavory gifts, these cannot be avoided on this earth. The question I ask is, now that I have this gift; What am I going to do with it? After much thought and in spite of pain it evoked, I was compelled to open it. Slowly, I tore away the wrappings and ribbons. I didn't want to touch them at first, but the fear of wrestling with these was worse than the reality. Finally, it was time to open the box. Did I

dare look into it? Would the inside be more of what I found on the outside? To my amazement, the contents of the package were beyond anything I experienced or immediately hoped to possess. For you see, the package contained precious jewels and metals. There was a bright gold nugget—it represented faith tested in the furnace and made stronger. In one corner was a cross of sterling silver. It reminded me that suffering was not in vain, rather, part of following Christ. The large, glittering diamond was a symbol of the resiliency one gains by weathering the tough times. The deep red ruby signified compassion— an orientation of reaching out to others and feeling with them. There was a pearl, perfectly round, that rolled from one side to the other. Immediately it reminded me of the 'roly-polies' that Ross (my six-year-old) sometimes brings into the house. I couldn't help but smile. With that smile I realized the pearl represented a sense of humor, the ability to see the light side of oneself and of life. Finally, there was a perfect emerald. Its deep green color is synonymous with growth and life.

"So you see, my friends, the real 'gifts' were inside the package. They were sent to me by a loving God. He probably offered these gifts to me at other times. However, I found them and learned to appreciate them in the face of death and suffering. And isn't our very faith such a paradox? For Jesus tells us it is in dying to ourselves that we find him and it is in dying to this life that we gain eternity.

"Every day, I thank God for the gift of another day. Each one is so precious. Also, I ask God to show me what he wants of me this day and ask him to help me to see everyone as he sees him/her. I am at peace inside walking with God. I look forward to 'better' days but with the knowledge that among them, will be scattered periods of further pain and suffering for that is the nature of life on this earth. As the saying goes, 'everything comes to pass, it doesn't come to stay.' "

IDA NEZEY, LAFAYETTE, LOUISIANA

Exactly two years from the day of my original diagnosis of breast cancer, I experienced what doctors refer to as an "abnormal exam." Abnormal as in "not quite normal" or abnormal as in "uh, oh . . . here we go again?", I asked, as the nurse started placing calls for an immediate MRI. That afternoon, the MRI confirmed the "abnormalities," not only in my original place of surgery but in a secondary location as well. "We'll do a mammogram," they said, and off I went for more testing. And more "abnormalities."

As I was being wheeled into surgery for a biopsy a few weeks later, I looked at my surgeon and said, "You know, cancer reminds me a lot of Arnold Schwarzenegger. It's powerful, it takes over the entire room when it enters, and you never know when it's going to say: **I'll be back**!" I was struggling with all of the emotions I had experienced two years before: anger, confusion, denial, and grief. But through it all, there surfaced one particular emotion that kept rising to the top that made it all possible, that helped to see me through: *hope.*

I realized that if I did have cancer again, I had what it takes to get through the process. I had the power of the letter "P." There was the power of people: my family, my friends, my staff and co-workers. There was the power of the physicians, and this time I knew them better, trusted them, knew how they operated. I had the power of prayer—that my faith could help me to understand why this was happening to me again. I had the power of my passion: to spread the word of joy and laughter despite the obstacles we all have in our everyday lives to overcome. But most importantly, the greatest "P" of all: I had the power of positive thinking.

The secret to a happy, joyful life is as simple as A, B, C . . .

Attitude is the key—be positive!

Believe in yourself—that you will get through your treatments.

Cheer others with your sunny disposition.

Donate your time to those less fortunate.

Eat dessert first!

Find a humor buddy to exchange jokes with.

Give the gift of laughter.

Ha ha, ho ho, hee hee.

Tickle your funny bone.

Invite your friends over for a celebration.

Join a support group.

Keep your spirits up.

Laugh at least twelve times daily!

Make a journal of all the funny experiences you have.

Nurse yourself with special treats every day.

Order something whimsical from a catalog.

Pursue a passion—something you've always wanted to do.

Quit that bad habit today!

Read a humorous book.

Smile at everyone you pass by.

Talk to an old friend you haven't heard from in ages.

Upbeat tapes and videos can cheer you.

Visit your relatives—even the ones who annoy you.

Write thank-you notes to your caregivers.

Xercise daily.

Yes I Can are words to repeat every day.

Zzzzz . . . get plenty of rest to be your best!

My biopsy came back benign. The experience only reinforced to me that every day, every moment is a gift to embrace, cherish and share. To all of us—the patients, survivors, family, friends, employers and caregivers who are living with cancer—never let go of the thing that makes getting up every day worth living for: the gift of hope.

CHAPTER VIII

How to Support a Friend or Loved One Who Has Cancer

They might not need me, but they might,
I'll let my head be just in sight;
A smile as small as mine might be
Precisely their necessity.
—EMILY DICKINSON

Don't ever be afraid to ask people for help. The love and support that people want to give you when you are diagnosed with cancer can absolutely get you through this experience on a day-by-day basis. Enclosed here you will find suggestions on how family and friends can pitch in and do something meaningful and worthwhile for you.

Complete with instructions to the cancer patient on how to accept the offers of assistance, these helpful hints are the "Martha Stewart" of cancer care for friends, family and caregivers worldwide. Simply hand out these suggestions when the voice on the other end of the phone says, "What can I do to help?"

None of us have any control over the timing of a diagnosis of cancer. As they say, "Cancer has its own calendar." If a friend or family member is given a diagnosis or has to go through surgery, treatment or hospitalization on or around a "special" day, plan to do something for them anyway to acknowledge the occasion despite their protests to the contrary. It will help take their mind off their situation, if even for only an hour or two. It will help them recognize that life must go on, and in the long run, they'll probably feel better just knowing you cared enough to remember.

To Cancer Patients

If you are going to the hospital, having a treatment, or just dealing with cancer on a special occasion, bring a little something to hand out to family, friends, physicians and caregivers to demonstrate your positive ATTITUDE. Bring blowers for New Year's or candy hearts for Valentine's Day, chocolates for Easter or balloons on your birthday. You can prove to everyone that you may be down, but you're not out!

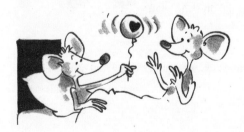

Laughter is the shortest distance between two people.

—ANONYMOUS

One of the "danger zones" for people with a diagnosis of cancer is when they tell you they don't want to see people or don't want to go out. Perhaps they don't feel well, or they are uncomfortable with their personal appearance. Make some special arrangements to take them out for an afternoon of lunch and a special activity: perhaps a funny movie matinee, or a walk in the park. Call ahead to the restaurant and request a private or secluded table where the two of you can talk. Make arrangements for some freshly cut flowers to be on the table or a cake to be delivered to celebrate the day. The cancer patient will forget their troubles for an afternoon and will be grateful that you still enjoy their company.

To Cancer Patients

If a friend or loved one offers to take you out for lunch or a special activity, take them up on their offer. It will take your mind off your treatments and current condition, and besides—it's lots of fun! You'll be glad you went!

We are all dependent on one another, every soul of us on earth.
—George Bernard Shaw

Facing surgery for cancer treatment can be as frightening for the caregiver of a cancer patient as it is for the patients themselves. Often the caregiver feels isolated, confused and unsure of what he/she can do in the situation. Organize a "comfort" party in the lobby area of the hospital on the day of the surgery. Invite family, friends, employers and neighbors to drop in and offer their support. Encourage people to bring food and beverages along with a guest book that can be signed with words of encouragement by the attendees that the caregiver can present to the cancer patient when they come out of surgery. 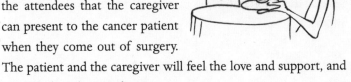 The patient and the caregiver will feel the love and support, and won't feel so alone in the experience.

To Cancer Patients

Ask a friend to offer support to your caregiver on the day of your surgery. You'll be comforted to know that there are people in the hospital rooting for you, and your loved one will be grateful for the support.

> *The last of the human freedoms—to choose one's attitude in any given set of circumstances, to choose one's own way.*
> —VICTOR FRANKL

A common reaction when you hear a friend or loved one has cancer is to volunteer to put the patient in touch with another friend or family member you know who has also faced the disease. While this can be comforting and supportive to talk to other people who have "been there; done that;" it can also be overwhelming to begin receiving calls from complete strangers.

Call the cancer patient first and offer to put them in touch with your other acquaintance. Then be sure to ask when a convenient time would be to call, and whether the patient would prefer to place the call themselves at their convenience or receive the call from your friend. Eventually the two will probably enjoy sharing their stories, but it is important that the timing be appropriate.

To Cancer Patients

Be assertive if you do not want to speak to strangers about your situation. Tell your friend or family member that you appreciate their concern and efforts to put you in touch with someone they know. Then let your friend know if you would, indeed, find comfort in speaking to someone else who has faced a diagnosis of cancer. You may make a new friend in the process!

Humor is the instinct for taking pain playfully.
—MAX EASTMAN

People going through cancer treatment often feel unattractive due to hair loss, weight changes, problems with their complexions or just not feeling "up to par." It's amazing what a compliment can do to lift one's spirits! Look the cancer patient in the eye and tell them they look *great*! Call attention to the positive changes or just the fact that the patient has made an effort to get out of the house to go to a movie or meet you for lunch. You'll be amazed at the positive reaction an encouraging word can bring. A smile on the face of a cancer patient will not only make their day . . . it will make yours, too!

To Cancer Patients

When someone gives you a compliment while you're going through your treatments, take it as an acknowledgment that you really are doing a great job! It takes an effort to get up and face each day when you don't feel well or have lost the confidence in your appearance. And remember, the changes are usually temporary. One day soon, it will all be behind you!

You can't really be strong until you see the funny side of things.
—KEN KESEY

Getting the proper rest and sleep is often a challenge for cancer patients. Fear and anxiety may cause sleepless nights; treatments may induce insomnia; pressures of chores and responsibilities may prevent a much-needed rest. Offer to "nap nanny"—come over to the cancer patient's house and do whatever needs to be done to allow for peace and quiet. If children or pets are a problem, offer to take them to your house for the day or night. If chores need to be done, come over and iron, cook, clean, or do yardwork while your friend rests comfortably. Bring a new pillow, a fresh set of sheets or a new pair of pajamas. Your friend or loved one will get some sleep, and you may find some time to dream, too!

To Cancer Patients

If you feel tired and run-down, ask a friend to help you find the time to take a nap. Give them a list of things they can do for you while you slumber. You'll wake up rested and refreshed, and they will feel great that they have been able to help. Sweet dreams!

In our whole life melody the music is broken off here and there by rests, and we foolishly think we have come to the end of time. God sends a time of forced leisure, a time of sickness and disappointed plans, and makes a sudden pause in the hymns of our lives. Be it ours to learn the time and not be dismayed at the rests.

—JOHN RUSKIN

Sitting through a chemotherapy treatment can be a lonely, long and depressing process for most cancer patients. Plan a "chemotherapy party" for the patient with two other friends. Offer to pick the patient up, drive them to their treatment, and spend the time doing something fun and unusual to get their mind off their current situation. Bring cards and play bridge or "500," rent a funny movie, pack a picnic basket with glasses for sparkling grape juice or bubbly 7-Up. All wear the same T-shirts or matching hats. The nurses and doctors will get a kick out of it, and all the other patients may join in your festivities! Your friend or loved one will feel the time whizzed by, and just think—another treatment over and done!

To Cancer Patients

Check to make sure your hospital or oncology clinic wouldn't mind if you brought visitors. Then pass the time with friends or family that you wouldn't (or couldn't) ordinarily spend time with. Your treatment will whiz by quickly, and who knows . . . you may have a lot of laughs!

There are three things which are real: God, human folly, and laughter. The first two are beyond our comprehension. So we must do what we can with the third.
—JOHN F. KENNEDY

Receiving a diagnosis of cancer is the most stressful time in someone's life, and most people don't know where to go or who to turn to. Visit your local library or bookstore and get one or two general books on cancer that will help explain the types of doctors your friend or loved one needs to see. Offer to help make calls to get referrals, and volunteer to call to make appointments. Drive the patient to their consultations and be available to help "take notes." Your friend or loved one will be grateful for the support and glad someone else had a "second pair of ears."

To Cancer Patients

Let a friend or loved one help you navigate the new and often frightening world of doctors, hospitals and clinics by allowing them to make some phone calls and drive you to your appointments. By asking them to record the doctor's comments, you will be grateful to have the notes to refer back to when you get home to sort things out.

*Laughter can relieve tension, soothe the
pain of disappointment and strengthen the spirit
for the formidable tasks that always lie ahead.*
—DWIGHT EISENHOWER

One of the most difficult and traumatic experiences faced by many cancer patients is the loss or thinning of hair during chemotherapy or radiation. Many patients are apprehensive of what they should do, or where they can go to buy scarves, hats, hairpieces or turbans. As a friend, make some phone calls in your area; talk to cancer clinics to find out where they recommend patients to go. Then make arrangements with your friend/family member to drive them to a wig salon or help make the phone call to an organization specializing in hair loss. Make a day of it—go to lunch or the park afterward. Your friend will appreciate your concern and support, and won't feel quite so "alone."

To Cancer Patients

Let your friends and family do some research for you and investigate the possibilities. You have enough on your mind already, and besides, it's always nice to get a second opinion on what looks best: the blond or brunette wig, the red or blue scarf. You'll be glad you brought a friend along!

There's nothing worth the wear of winning,
But laughter and the love of friends.
—HILLAIRE BELLOC

The thought of cooking a meal at the end of the day after having chemotherapy or radiation can send even the most positive cancer patient into a downward spiral. Most patients are either too tired, too nauseous, or too preoccupied to think about buying groceries, slaving over the stove and setting a table. Offer to prepare a meal for the cancer patient. Contact several mutual friends and set up a "schedule" so the cancer patient has a meal delivered one, two, even three times a week. Include some "special touches" like a bouquet of flowers, a copy of your recipe, or some colorful paper napkins. The cancer patient is insured of a nutritious meal, the "muss and fuss" is minimal, and the gratitude is forever.

To Cancer Patients

When someone offers to make you a meal—take them up on their offer. Your friends and family want to help you, and this is a way that they can shine! Everyone will outdo themselves with their favorite recipe. You can eat like a king or queen, and besides: the leftovers can carry you for days!

Enjoy.

Happiness is good health and a bad memory.
—INGRID BERGMAN

A common reaction of people who hear someone they know has cancer is to pull away or avoid the cancer patient because they simply don't know what to say. Worse yet, they don't want to say the wrong thing, so often times, they don't say anything. Any gesture of friendship and recognition of the disease is welcome: from a simple card or call, to a gift of flowers, the words "I care about you, and I'm thinking of you" is a day brightner for any cancer patient.

To Cancer Patients

If a person you know seems to be avoiding you since you received your diagnosis, don't think they have deserted you— they just may not have the right words to say. Next time you see them, let them know that you've missed hearing from them and hope they will keep in touch. Your gesture will put them at ease and let them know you're doing "OK!"

> *The most utterly lost of all days is that*
> *in which you have not once laughed.*
> —SEBASTIAN ROCH CHAMFORT

Visual stimulation can go a long way toward improving our outlook on life. If someone you know is having cancer surgery, bring some brightly colored or decorated sheets to cover their hospital bed. Disney sheets or animated cartoon characters can cheer anyone's spirit. Bring some pictures of loved ones to put by the bedside along with a beautifully painted water vase and cup. The bright colors and unusual decor will not only bring a smile to the patient, but the staff at the hospital may make themselves at home, too!

To Cancer Patients

As long as you are going to be in the hospital for a few days (or weeks, as the case may be), make yourself at home. Ask friends or loved ones to bring some of your favorite things from home (a favorite stuffed animal, pillow or blanket). The familiar atmosphere will cheer you up and remind you that soon you will be back at "home sweet home"!

A keen sense of humor helps us
overlook the unbecoming, understand
the unconventional, tolerate the
unpleasant, overcome the unexpected and
outlast the unbearable.
—BILLY GRAHAM

When summer arrives, the thought of doing yardwork in the heat and humidity can be overwhelming to most cancer patients. Offer to set up a "pool" of friends to take turns weeding, watering, and working in their yard and/or patio area. Plant some brightly colored annuals to bring daily cheer to the cancer patient. Place some decorative yard ornaments and buy a special watering can. The site of a well manicured yard will not only bring a smile to the patient, but who knows . . . they may offer to join you in the fun!

To Cancer Patients

Prepare a list of tasks in your yard or patio you'd like to have completed of things that seem too overwhelming. Pick out some colors and types of flowers that bring a smile to your face. Then offer to serve the lemonade and cookies as your friends do what they like to do best: *help you!*

An effort made for the happiness of others lifts us above ourselves.
—L. M. CHILD

If a friend or loved one is going into the hospital for cancer surgery, bring a Walkman and some favorite tapes for them to listen to. Music can help relax the patient and take their mind off the upcoming surgery. Post operation it can soothe their anxieties and perhaps help them fall asleep. The patient will appreciate your gesture and may even hum or sing along!

To Cancer Patients

Jot down the names of a few of your favorite musicians or bands and give them to a friend who wants to help. Friends and family are anxious to do something helpful, and you may end up with a wonderful collection of your favorite music to enjoy for many years to come.

> *Laughter is a melody, a concert for the heart.*
> *A tickling by the angels, creating living art.*
> *Laughter heals and comforts,*
> *It's sometimes gentle, sometimes bold.*
> *Laughter is a freeing dance performed within*
> *the soul.*
> —SERENE W. WEST

A real day brightener for any cancer patient is receiving mail—a note, a card, an article that lets them know you are thinking about them. Write a "Thank You" note to your friend or family member who has cancer that tells them how much you appreciate their friendship. Thank them for the different things they have done to bring joy and laughter into your life. Remind them of some little gesture they did that made *your* day. The patient will savor the memories and will most certainly feel loved and thought of for the rest of the day.

To Cancer Patients

Design a simple "Thank You" note of your own that you can return to friends and family members who do something special for you. Here's one written by a special friend of The Cancer Club®:

For all your good wishes and candy
The balloons and stuffed animals were dandy.
Contributions, beautiful flowers, gourmet meals
and games—It's hard to keep track of all the names.
Cards, books, visits, calls on the phone
Gave strength to me, I was not alone.
Your hopes and prayers are appreciated more
than I can say—Hopes and dreams for a brighter day.
Many Thanks!

We all know how inviting and comforting the feel of a newly aired bed feels. The thought of changing sheets, doing laundry and making the bed may seem overwhelming to a cancer patient. Offer to come over daily/weekly/or even once a month to fluff the pillows and keep the sheets and covers smooth. Purchase a special pillow to help prop the patient for reading or watching TV. Add the sound of trickling water with a small fountain and make sure fresh flowers in the bedroom are receiving their needed dose of water. The cancer patient will be snug as a bug in a rug and will sleep better, too!

To Cancer Patients

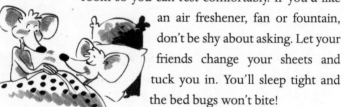

Let your friend or family member pamper you in your own room so you can rest comfortably. If you'd like an air freshener, fan or fountain, don't be shy about asking. Let your friends change your sheets and tuck you in. You'll sleep tight and the bed bugs won't bite!

A good laugh and a long sleep are the two best cures.
—IRISH PROVERB

On a friend or family member's first day of treatment (chemotherapy or radiation), make arrangements to have a single flower
delivered to the facility where the treatment will take place. On
day two, have two flowers delivered; day three, three flowers and
so on until, on the last day of treatment send a full bouquet of
flowers and balloons. Your friend or family member will delight
in the experience. The staff members will be sure to get involved,
and the other patients in the waiting area will smile in appreciation of the beauty and all the attention.

To Cancer Patients

Be sure to let your family members and friends know the
phone number and address of your treatment facility so they can
reach you and offer you cheer. Have your hospital or clinic xerox
business cards with their location information and write a small
note, "come visit me sometime." You'll be surprised how many
visitors you may find will come help pass the time away during
those regular visits for treatment.

Heaven isn't a place . . . it's a feeling.
—AUTHOR UNKNOWN

We all know how much it means to receive good wishes and thoughts from loved ones and friends, but someone facing cancer may feel overwhelmed by the need to respond to others' gestures of caring. Offer to keep a journal or log of cards, meals, flowers and gifts. Buy a box of notecards or postcards and have them preprinted with a word of thanks. Allow the patient to add a few words of their own, then stamp, address and take them to the post office. The patient will feel relieved that they are responding to others' friendship, and you will provide a very valuable service to all.

To Cancer Patients

Ask a close friend or family member to help you with your thank-yous when needed. Let them know what kind of stationery you like (flowers, animals, cartoons, sports, etc.) and send them to the drugstore for cards and stamps. Let them update your holiday mailing list while they address envelopes for you. You'll feel satisfied that you are responding to people's gestures of love, and your "helper" will feel great knowing they've helped *you!*

The head thinks, the hands labor, but it is the heart that laughs!
—LIZ CURTIS-HIGGS

It can be comforting to have a special relative or loved one come visit us when we're going through cancer treatments. Make arrangements for that "special someone" (sister, brother, college roommate, etc.) to come for a visit. If possible, purchase an airline ticket to help defray the costs. Make arrangements to pick the visitor up from the airport and have them stay with you if the cancer patient doesn't have room at their place. Remind them to bring old photos and stories of days gone by. Then plan some simple, quiet get-togethers where the "old friends/family" can exchange memories, stories and spend the day in laughter. You will have provided the gift of a lifetime, and the memories will remain forever.

To Cancer Patients

If it's been a long time since you've seen that "special someone" in your life, let your friends know how much it would mean to you to share some valuable time together. Give your friends the phone number/address/E-mail address of your friend or loved one and ask them to get in touch with your special loved one for you. You may just end up with a surprise guest that will boost your spirits and bring a smile to your face. That's what friends are for!

Laughter loves company even more than misery loves company!
—JOEL GOODMAN, PH.D.

I am often asked "What can I do for my dear friend (relative, loved one) with cancer?" One of the most important days in the life of any cancer patient is that infamous *last day of treatment*. Whether it's the final treatment of radiation therapy or the very last chemotherapy, the day is anticipated with a mixture of joy, accomplishment, relief, sadness and fear.

Mark *your* calendar and make a point of contacting the cancer patient to congratulate them and wish them well. A call, a card, or a bottle of champagne can go a long way toward telling your friend

"You Did It!"

To Cancer Patients

Let your friends and family in on your final days of treatments. It's a day that will remain etched in your mind for many years to come. It's a grand accomplishment!

There's no thrill in easy sailing
When the skies are clear and blue,
There's no joy in merely doing
*   things*
Which anyone can do.
But there is some satisfaction
that is mighty sweet to take,
When you reach a destination that
You thought you'd never make.
—SPIRELLA

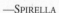

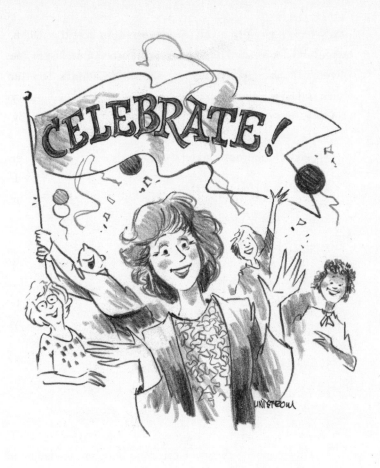

I truly hope I have given you some suggestions here that will be helpful and appreciated by all parties concerned. But, just in case I haven't, I am prepared. Below, "Christine Clifford's Top Ten Quick and Easy Things You Can Do to Bring Joy and Laughter to Cancer Patients":

10. Send a humorous card for a change.

9. Send a cookie bouquet.

8. Rent a funny movie.

7. Share a funny story.

6. Give a funny book.

5. Send a painted coconut telegram. (The one I send reads, "Go nuts. Get healthy!")

4. Tell a joke.

3. Create a humor basket.

2. Send a cartoon.

And the number 1 thing you can do to bring joy and laughter to cancer patients . . .

1. Shave *your* head in sympathy!

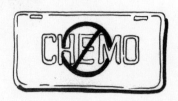

CHAPTER IX

And If the End Is Drawing Near . . .

I think that wherever your journey takes you, there are new gods waiting there, with divine patience—and laughter.
—SUSAN WATKINS

"I have always had a sense of humor and have raised my three grown girls to have a sense of humor, too. When I was going through treatment, I told my girls I have a way to let them know I am around after I die.

"I told them that I will make their noses itch. That way they will know it is 'me.' They laughed and said, 'Mom, we all have allergies; our noses always itch.' I replied, 'Yeah, but after I die, it will be me.'

"This way I have planted the seed and every time they itch their noses, they will think of me and know that Mom is still bugging them even after death.

"Laugh a lot and keep on moving!"
MADELINE DAVIDSON, OMAHA, NEBRASKA

Alas, we all have to go sometime. So when we do, I hope we can do it with a good sense of humor.

Unfortunately, death is inevitable for each of us. However, our ability to maintain a good sense of humor until the end is perhaps the greatest privilege of all: the ability to laugh even in the face of death.

Life is a gift—one more truly appreciated by those who have faced a diagnosis of cancer. Did you wake up this morning and embrace the day? I did, and it's something that cancer taught me to do. I didn't always have this appreciation for life—living was something I simply took for granted. Cancer allowed me to realize that every day is a gift to be cherished.

Today is our gift. Shake the box; unwrap it slowly. Touch, smell, hear and taste the makings of our day. Enjoy it; savor it; and embrace it. Ultimately, time is all we have and the idea isn't to save it, but to savor it . . .

"Mary Jane, a sixteen-year-old, vivacious, fun-loving and outgoing girl was diagnosed with cancer intertwining her esophagus and other organs. Due to recurrence, three times Mary Jane underwent chemo, each time losing her hair. Sometimes with a ball cap, sometimes with bare head, Mary Jane greeted friends and visitors to her room. One time going home Mary Jane, her hair barely a half inch long, as usual, *journeyed to the mall to be with her friends. At the mall someone who had not seen her recently said, 'Wow! What a neat haircut! What's it called?' Mary Jane cooly said, 'It's called a chemo-cut!' Unperturbed, the other person asked, 'And where do you get it?' Without losing a beat, Mary Jane said, 'Oh, God gives it!' Mary Jane lost her battle with cancer, seventeen years of age—a very beautiful person."*

Father Bob Striegel university of iowa hospital, ottumwa, iowa

"My wife died a year ago as a result of pancreatic cancer. Prior to that she had had two mastectomies about nine years apart. I want to testify to the truth of humor, healing and coping. I am a retired Episcopal priest.

"My wife had taken her wig to the beauty shop. She'd always intended to get it restyled. When the operator was finished, she was trying it on and an old friend came in and said, 'Oh, Beryl, your hair looks so beautiful.' She replied, 'Well, it should; it cost enough!' "

Tom Cooper, camillus, new york

Life Line

Be sure to get a mammogram,
The screening test for breast cancer;
You may not become a MILLIONAIRE,
But that is my FINAL ANSWER!

Joan T. Muller, vero beach, florida

"While our ten year-old daughter, Kara, endured a four-year-long battle with both non-Hodgkin's lymphoma and A.L.L. leukemia, our family felt blessed when reasons for laughter came our way. On one such occasion, we were on what would be our last family vacation

when Kara became very ill and was admitted to a large medical center in Sacramento, California. After getting settled into her room, the nurses insisted that she order a lunch that would be made special for her. Kara pondered the menu choices and finally decided on a deluxe hamburger complete with cheese and all the trimmings. It seemed like an eternity to her before her long-awaited meal was finally delivered. She removed the plate cover that was keeping her meal warm during transit and immediately began to laugh. Upon investigation, we found that she had a delicious-looking bun but no meat or trimmings. What began as a mistake in the kitchen, ended up giving one very ill little girl and her family a reason to laugh. Kara lost her battle, but to this day, when life throws us a curve, we refer to life as a hamburger with no meat in it."

BILL AND CHARLOTTE HAWKINS, TYGH VALLEY, OREGON

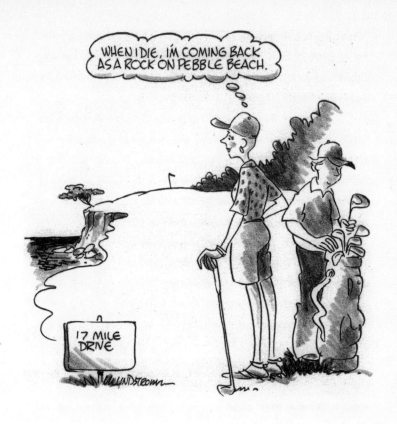

"My father-in-law, who was dying of brain cancer, came home from one of his hospital stays. It was his and my mother-in-law's wedding anniversary so I suggested that they invite a few friends over for dinner and I would make a turkey.

"Jimmy managed to get out of bed to join us. He enjoyed the meal but the strain of feeding himself and the presence of guests were obviously tiring him. Noticing this, and knowing that he could not hear very well, my mother-in-law wrote a note and passed it to me to give to him. I read it and got hysterical with laughter. She remembered what she just wrote and laughed out loud, too.

"The note said, 'Happy Anniversary, dear. Do you want to go to bed?'

"Jimmy read what his wife had written, looked up across the table, and with a twinkle in his eye and a smile on his face said to her, 'I would love to dear, but we have company.'

"It was only a brief moment of levity in his difficult last months but it was a moment that was retold at his memorial service and long remembered after he was gone."

ALLEN KLEIN, SAN FRANCISCO, CALIFORNIA

"You know what they say about them stem cells . . . here today, gone to marrow."

JIM RICHARDS, JOLIET, ILLINOIS

"A few days after hearing about the birth of a new baby cousin, Dana (age five) and her mother were driving home from the grocery store. Dana suddenly became very thoughtful and asked, 'Mommy, why does God make people born alive, when they all die later, anyway?' Her mother had to think very quickly after such a philosophical question, but finally attempted an answer: 'Perhaps,' she said, 'God wants to give us time to do good things while we're here on earth.' 'Oh,' Dana replied—with a twinkle in her eye, 'like stopping for some Dunkin' Donuts?' "

JANET M. WEISS, MINNEAPOLIS, MINNESOTA

"When my wife's medullary thyroid cancer spread to her bones in late 1993 the prognosis was for no more than five years. It turned out to be three and a half. During that time I wrote free verse poetry, chronicling the emotion-filled story of our journey. I continued to write after she died and a year later was encouraged to put my writing into a book for sharing. It was a totally new experience for me so I ended up hiring a small publisher to steer me through the project. Since I was paying all of the bills, cost was significant. I had enlisted the aid of my youngest daughter, Laura, to help me evaluate the publisher I had chosen before I signed any contract. Laura was so very close to her mother, sharing an adult-to-adult closeness and spirituality that was marvelous to see. So when I made the decision to proceed I called Laura in Chicago and told her of my plan.

   "I covered a few of the final details, casually mentioning the fact that the book would be in softcover. This is what is most often done with a first-time author and this type of book. It was recommended strongly by the publisher since hardcover with dust jacket would be twice the cost to me. Well, there was a pause in the phone connection at that point. Then Laura, true to her mother's spirit, uttered four words that changed my book, a book that changed my life. She simply said, 'Dad, Mom deserves hardcover.' There was silence while I digested her words. But it took only a few seconds for the lightbulb to go on and for me to say, 'You're right.' My hardcover book, Through Death to Life, is a beautiful tribute to my wife, Patty. The wraparound book jacket features a spectacular sunrise picture and some moving endorsements, displaying the dignity and class of Laura's mother. I will always be thankful that Laura spoke important words from her heart and that I listened."

RON GRIES, BLOOMFIELD HILLS, MICHIGAN

"I was diagnosed with inflammatory breast cancer metastasized to bones. As a single mother of three boys, the sadness felt was for them. We've gotten through the seven months with God, smile therapy, pretending to be healthy by dancing and singing to keep happy juices flowing and the lymph system moving.

"Just yesterday I was reassuring my eighteen-year-old that if possible, even if I died I'd always be there to listen to him. He responded abruptly, 'Sorry, Mom, hold it right there. I will pay you to rest in peace. I know your intentions are good but I can't be worried about you hanging out in my Christmas tree, whispering in my ear, inhabiting my closet or hiding under my bed.' I said, 'Son, I would never in my life scare you!' 'We're not talking life here, Mom—we're talking death. Believe me, you've given me the skills to cope, I can handle the grief, and I can wait until the time comes to see you again. How much do you want to promise not to haunt me? I can't be living my life looking over my shoulder, wondering what you're up to now.' So much for reassurance. Thanks for letting me share."

CLARE SHEA, WEST PALM BEACH, FLORIDA

The Future

This week, my surgeon called one night
To talk about the poem I didn't write.

We agreed that everyone has done their best.
There is, however, no guarantee.

It is enough, I said, that today
I'm fully alive and cancer free.

Is it less of a miracle if it lasts only a year or two?
I know my answer,
What about you?

DEBORAH TRENEER PITMAN, RICHLAND, WASHINGTON

Afterglow

I'd like the memory of me to be a happy one.
I'd like to leave an afterglow of smiles
    when life is done.
I'd like to leave an echo
    whispering softly down the ways.
Of happy times and laughing times
    and bright and sunny days.
I'd like the tears of those who grieve
    to dry before the sun.
Of happy memories that I leave
    when life is done.

—AUTHOR UNKNOWN

Don't Forget To Laugh™

I look around the chemo room,
Watch doctors, and their staff,
And saddened faces, then I think,
"Don't forget to laugh."

It isn't easy sitting here,
It's hard to stand the gaff
Of needles sticking everywhere.
"Don't forget to laugh."

Some folks will try a great big smile.
It comes out only half.
So why not just go all the way.
"Don't forget to laugh."

When chemo hurts you quite a bit
A nice long drink you quaff,
And like our English friends would say,
"Don't forget to lawff."

Standing there at heaven's gate,
St. Pete with mighty staff,
Will say as I am welcomed in,
"Don't forget to laugh."

He'll say, "A cure for cancer's found.
The whole thing, not just half."
Then with a real un-saintly wink,
"Don't forget to laugh."

EDWARD J. BECKWELL, ST. CLAIR SHORES, MICHIGAN

"I belong to a support group that meets twice a year for a camping weekend in April and September. One young man who had cancer was told he had six months to live. He was in a wheelchair, on oxygen and chemo often. The nurses at the hospital got several members of our support group involved and talked him into coming to camp. Everyone gave him huge warm greetings. We visited him at home, took foods and showed someone cared.

"The men took turns picking him up to attend birthday suppers and our Christmas party. He lived almost three years. His doctor said he thrived on the love he received from those of us around him. Someone called each day. At times, more than one person called. He kept count of his phone calls and visits. He wrote poetry about how nicely he was changed.

"One time at camp, three men lifted him into a paddle boat and paddled all around the lake. James Putt passed away about one and a half years ago. He went to a birthday fish fry, ate over three dozen shrimp, got sick and was hospitalized before morning. Believe me, he died happy.

"People make a difference. Love and caring can change our lives. The doctors called this a miracle."

EDNA P. GRESKO, RED BAY, ALABAMA

My husband John's favorite aunt Nancy died of lung cancer several years ago. I was deeply touched by the eulogy her best friend, Anne, read at her funeral:

"I first met Nancy back in high school. It was in a record store on Ninth Street right off Nicollet. I can still see her as clearly as if it were yesterday. She was, to put it simply, absolutely beautiful, and I thought, 'I wonder if she is nice or will she be stuck up and vain or "what"?' Well, 'what' turned out to be one of the most wonderful gifts

I have ever received, my friendship with Nancy. Over the years we have shared good and bad times together, lots of parties, lots of hockey games, just plain living, if you will, and it was great. But it wasn't until the day I moved into the same apartment complex nine and a half years ago that something quite miraculous occurred. I discovered I had a friend who loved me unconditionally. That friendship blossomed and grew and was treated with great care by both of us. I could not believe how lucky I was.

"We had been in our apartment about ten days when the phone rang one evening, rather late. This voice said, 'Meet me in the stairwell with a nightcap, right now!' 'But Nancy, I'm ready to go to bed!' And she replied, 'So?' With my husband, Jack, shaking his head, off I went with drink in hand to the beginning of the unfolding of a whole new world of so much laughter and fun, like the times when girls are young and spend hours sharing everything with their 'best' friend.

"Seven years ago I had some cancer surgery. It was unexpected and frightening. One night in the hospital, the phone rang, and it was Nancy. I burst into tears and with that Nancy was off and running chattering on about this and that, asking me to be very explicit over why I was crying, and comforting me like a mother does to a child. We talked for quite a while and when we hung up I felt secure and happy again. About twenty-five minutes later, now close to 9:30 P.M., I heard a little tap at my door. It opened and a hand was thrust in holding a chocolate sundae with a cherry on top. Behind that hand was Nancy with her wonderful smile, a big hug, an act of love I'll never forget.

"Nancy was like no other person I have ever met. She was a free spirit, embracing life with such gusto. As if she couldn't get enough of it. She laughed and danced her way into all our hearts. She wore her bright clothes and wonderously junky jewelry with great panache. She never ever said an unkind word about anyone. She'd be riding in a go-cart when all of a sudden, she would throw her arms up to the sky,

*laughing that wonderful laugh and say, 'Oh, this is so much fun!' And
I would think, 'This is one wonderful woman!'*

"*See you in the stairwell . . .*"

ANNE EASTMAN, MINNEAPOLIS, MINNESOTA, IN MEMORY OF NANCY JENKINS

> *I have no yesterdays,*
> *Time took them away;*
> *Tomorrow may not be—*
> *But I have Today.*
> —PEARL YEADON MCGINNIS

I hope we all meet in the stairwell together some day.

Having been diagnosed with cancer at the age of forty, I used to worry "what if I only live another year, three years, five years?" Now my optimism has me asking, "What if I've only lived half of my life? What will I do with another forty years?" Well, I may not live another forty years, but I know what I'll do with whatever time I have left on this earth.

I will meet people wherever I go. Have you made a new friend lately? I will read and study and educate myself. Have you learned something new this week? I will set new goals of things I want to accomplish—this week, this month, this year. Have you set a goal to get through your treatments, celebrate your survival anniversary, help a friend in need? I will laugh every day. Have you told a joke, heard an amusing story, read a funny book?

Today is the perfect time for new beginnings. Begin living, loving, and laughing *today*! And oh, by the way, don't forget to laugh!™

Epilogue

I have learned many, many things in my seven-year journey with cancer. But the thing I've learned the most is that everyone who has cancer is a hero. Each of you has a story to share, and if we could take the time to read all of your stories, every one of them would pull at our heartstrings if we let them.

My story is no different than any of yours. I'm just very blessed, grateful to all of you for reading about my story, and I'd like to leave you with a poem I wrote:

Laughter: Prescription for a Cure

My life was perfect, or so it seemed
It far surpassed what I had dreamed
My boys were healthy, ages twelve and nine
My twenty-year marriage was doing fine
I had more friends than I could see
For a brand-new house, I held the key

I'd cracked that "glass ceiling" for which I had fought
Life doesn't get better than this, I thought.

One day without warning a lump appeared
It can't be the thing that so deeply I feared
I knew as I drove to the doctor that noon
My life would be changing profoundly and soon
A biopsy was done right on the spot
They hoped it was early, this lump I had caught
The wait for results was frightening and long
What had I done for my life to go wrong?

I'll never forget that one day in December
The words as he spoke them I hardly remember
"You have cancer" he said, his words rang in my ears
And before I could stop, I cried buckets of tears
The anger, confusion, denial and grief
To die and escape would seem such a relief
Then I looked all around me, the things that I had
To fight and continue could not be that bad.

I tackled my treatments like nobody could
I did everything specialists told me I should
Friends, family, employers all gave me support
Yet despite all their gestures, I felt something was short
I realized that laughter was just what I need
And once that I found it, I planted the seed
It may not cure cancer or other disease
But it will take your mind off and give it a tease.

So if you're a patient, survivor or friend
And you want to help win that race in the end
Remember that ATTITUDE is the key to success
A good one can do it for you, is my guess
So nothing is ever quite perfect, it seems
Our lives take many turns and often sway from our dreams
Look around and rejoice in the things that you have
Oh yes, one last reminder . . . don't forget to laugh!™

People are the only creatures on earth
who can celebrate the joy of being alive.

—CHRISTINE CLIFFORD

Have You Heard?

Sometimes the most helpful and practical items for cancer patients come from the creativity and experience of cancer patients themselves. Enclosed here please find a list of resources, often created by cancer patients, that we've found very useful and comforting.

ABOUT . . . Books?

The following books and/or booklets have been written by some of the contributors you have read in this book:

Bald in the Land of Big Hair (a true story) by Joni Rodgers, Harper Collins Publishers, New York, NY, 2000, 253 pages, $24.00. Bookstores.

Can You Come Here Where I Am? The Poetry and Prose of Seven Breast Cancer Survivors by The Write-Away Group (including author Rita Busch), E.M. Press, Inc., Manassas, VA, 1998, 222 pages, $21.95. (800) 727-4630.

The Courage to Laugh: Humor, Hope and Healing in the Face of Death and Dying by Allen Klein, Jeremy P. Tarcher/Putnam, 1998, 220 pages, $14.95. www.allenklein.com

Duck Soup for the Diehard Soul: Double Spice for Disabled Soles by Crockett Lane Grabbe (under the pen name of SeaLane

Gray), Lightning Source Press and lst-books.com (Ebook), 2001, 100 pages, $11.95. (800) 839-8640. www.lst books.com

The Healing Power of Humor by Allen Klein, Jeremy P. Tarcher/ Putnam, 1989, 216 pages, $12.95. www.allenklein.com

The Luckiest Unlucky Man Alive by Bill Goss, BookWorld Press, Inc., Sarasota, FL., 1998, 211 pages, $14.95. 1-800-444-2524.

Pinky Swear: The Gift of a Lifetime by Dawn M. Chicilo, Tree-House Ink, North Oaks, MN, 2000, 151 pages, $16.95. www.treehouseink.com

Through Death to Life by Ron Gries, Proctor Publications, LLC, Ann Arbor, Michigan, 1999, 237 pages, $22.00. 1-800-343-3034.

Triumphs of the Human Spirit: Real Cancer Survivors, Real Battles, Real Victories by Barry W. Summers, Writers Club Press, an imprint of iUniverse, Inc., Lincoln, NE, 2001, 182 pages, $13.95. www.iuniverse.com.

Well Versed in Cancer by Deborah Treneer Pitman, Lourdes Health Network, Pasco, WA, October 7, 1997. The funds from the sale of this booklet support *Generation Us* for women who cannot afford cancer treatment. $10.00 donation requested. (509) 542-3055.

ABOUT . . . Organizations?

The following organizations have shown to provide comfort and assistance to cancer patients:

Chemo Angels: Dedicated to adding a ray of sunshine to the lives of those undergoing treatment for cancer. You will be "adopted" by a Chemo Angel who, through small gifts, cards, notes, etc., will support and encourage you during the course of your treatment. To be "adopted" or to become an "Angel" volunteer, visit www.chemoangels.com or write P.O. Box 1971, Julian, CA 92036.

First Connection: Sponsored by The Leukemia and Lymphoma Society. This program matches recently diagnosed patients with people who've experienced leukemia or a similar cancer. These peer survivors offer more than hope and empathy; they're also trained in counseling. For information, call (800) 955-4572.

The Friend's Health Connection: This group will introduce you to someone with a similar cancer by phone, E-mail, or regular mail. Call (800) 48-FRIEND or write P.O. Box 114, New Brunswick, NJ 08903.

The National Coalition for Cancer Survivorship: Living with cancer is a battle no one should have to fight alone. To combat the isolation many people feel after being diagnosed, this group offers a toll-free number to get information about treatment, employment, and insurance issues, as well as emotional support. All calls are confidential and requested information will be mailed at no charge. Call 888-937-6227.

ABOUT . . . Spiritual Support?

The Joyful Noiseletter: This delightful newsletter from the Fellowship of Merry Christians is full of jokes, anecdotes, cartoons and more in their ministry to spread joy and good cheer. Published monthly, they also have a catalog of books, prints, and cassettes with a focus on Christian joy, humor and celebration. Call 1-800-877-2757.

ABOUT . . . Organizations for Children?

Kids Cancer Network: Visit www.kidscancernetwork.org for an organization committed to children fighting cancer and their families.

Kids Konnected: Providing "friendship, understanding, education and support for kids who have a parent with cancer," this organization offers a newsletter, a Teddy Bear and more. Call (800) 899-2866 or visit www.kidskonnected.org.

Kidscope: A nonprofit organization whose purpose is to create and provide educational materials to help children cope with changes in the family when a parent has cancer. Kidscope provides free videotapes (available in Spanish and Arabic) and special comic books for children (available in Spanish). Call (404) 233-0001, or write Kidscope, c/o 3399 Peachtree Road, Suite 2020, Atlanta, GA 30326.

ABOUT . . . Products?

Cancer Ed: Helping Children Understand Cancer: This user friendly video (*My Hair's Falling Out . . . Am I Still Pretty?*) and workbook (*Things Change All the Time . . . When Someone You Know Has Cancer*) are designed to connect students and teachers, schools, families and communities. Call (800) 221-3170.

Conversations!: The newsletter for those fighting ovarian cancer. Free subscription. Call (806) 355-2565 or visit www.ovarian-news.org.

Eating Hints for Cancer Patients Before, During and After Treatment: To order this booklet or other patient education materials, call the Cancer Information Service, a program of the National Cancer Institute at (800) 4-CANCER.

ECAP (Exceptional Cancer Patients) Insights, The Official Newsletter: Started by Bernie Siegel, this informative and motivational biannual publication is a charitable organization. To subscribe and become an ECAP Angel, call (800) 861-3296.

Friends For Life?: To obtain a free copy of this delightful book by cancer survivor Elizabeth Mertens Yaeger call (414) 291-1736 and leave your name and address. Or write Mary Ann Lorentz, Oncology Outreach RN, St. Mary's Hospital, 2323 N. Lake Drive, Milwaukee, WI 53211.

Guide to Complementary and Alternative Cancer Methods from the American Cancer Society. (888) 227-5552 or www.cancer.org.

I Remember You: A Grief Journal: by Laynee Wild. Helps you overcome the loss of a loved one. (800) 242-7737.

Janelle! Hats, etc: Provides soft headware and bangs for those suffering from hair loss: stylish, non-therapeutic hats, sleep caps and more. Visit them on the Web at www.janelle-hats.com or call 877-396-4287.

Karing—A Patient's Pal?: A complete way to organize medical information, therapy plans, medicines, and expenses, this special binder was created by a young cancer patient's mother. 1-800-9 KARING.

Keys to Health: A three-CD set designed for your well-being. "Paul Gilman is a modern-day Beethoven" says ABC News about this collection. "Letting Go," "Healing Waters" and "Sensual Surroundings" are meant to celebrate, console and heal. To order call 1-800-468-6333 or visit www.keystohealth.com ($24.95 plus $4.95 shipping/handling). Music is good medicine.

Shadow Buddies: These delightful dolls offer a positive opportunity to communicate and educate people about cancer and other conditions. They also make great pads to protect the chest area following surgery, or provide a fun way to collect autographs of all your friends that have helped you along the way. Choose from "Oncology Buddy," "HIV/Aids Buddy," "Survivor Buddy" and more. For further information, call 1-888-BUDDIE 1.

Tessin's Night Sweats Linens: Invented by a cancer survivor who was thrown into menopause following chemotherapy, these cotton terry velour pillowcases and sheet covers will keep you dry and comfortable all night long. (800) 480-8608. www. tessin.net. Don't sweat it!

The Healing Way: A Journal for Cancer Survivors: This structured journal helps cancer patients and survivors write about their life—a healing experience. (781) 944-9553 or www.writingto heal.com. (2000 by Element Books, Boston).

The Lung Cancer Manual: A comprehensive publication to guide those with lung cancer developed by the Alliance for Lung Cancer Advocacy, Support and Education (ALCASE). For information, call (800) 298-2436.

You've Just Been Told You Have Cancer: This fifty-minute video will help you ask the right questions and make informed decisions regarding your medical and emotional care. Included with video is a fifty-six-page guidebook and Cancer Resources List. (800) 401-2233 from Life Care Concepts, Inc.

Victoria's Quilts: Handmade quilts made by volunteer quilters are donated to cancer patients or treatment facilities. The purpose of the quilts is to make the cancer patients a little warmer and a little more comfortable. For information on receiving or making a quilt, call (310) 937-2508 or E-mail victoriasquilts @hotmail.com.

ABOUT . . . Web Sites?

www.cancerclub.com provides humorous and helpful products for people with cancer. Books, audiocassettes, videotapes, PC software, custom jewelry and more. Subscribe to a quarterly newsletter and join The Cancer Club® today. Don't forget to laugh!™

www.cancerfatigue.org provides information about the extreme exhaustion that often accompanies cancer treatments. Fatigue affects 76 percent of cancer patients and is one of the least understood side effects. Hosted by the Oncology Nursing Society.

www.cancernews.com is dedicated to bringing patients and their families the latest information on cancer diagnosis, treatment and prevention.

www.canceronline.org helps put some control back into the lives of cancer patients and their families by providing access to clinical information for all kinds of cancers and practical support and encouragement on a wide variety of topics.

www.cardblvd.com helps bring cheer by sending greeting cards for all occasions.

www.sharedexperience.org provides an open collection of firsthand accounts by cancer patients and their caregivers.

www.ulmanfund.org provides support programs, education and resources to benefit young adults who are affected by cancer, and to promote awareness and prevention of cancer.

Bibliography

Armstrong, Lance. *It's Not about the Bike—My Journey Back to Life*, G. P. Putnam's Sons, New York, NY, 2000.

Berk, L. S. & S. A. Tan, "Immune System Changes During Humor Associated with Laughter," *Clinical Research*. (39), 1991, 124A.

Cousins, Norman. *Anatomy of an Illness*, W. W. Norton, New York, NY, 1979.

Nielson, Dr. Jerri. *Ice Bound: A Doctor's Incredible Battle for Survival at the South Pole*, Talk Miramax Books, 2001.

Simonton, D. Carl, M.D., Stephanie M. Simonton and James Creighton. *Getting Well Again: A Step by Step Guide to Overcoming Cancer*, Bantam Books, New York, NY, 1978.

About the Author

Before her bout with breast cancer, **Christine Clifford** had definitely cracked the glass ceiling. At the age of forty, she was senior vice president for SPAR Marketing Services, an international information and merchandising services firm in Minneapolis, Minnesota.

Once the top salesperson in the billion dollar service industry, Christine was responsible for accounts with Kmart, Toy "Я" Us, Procter & Gamble, AT&T, Tyco Toys and L'Oreal, among others.

Diagnosed with breast cancer in December of '94, Christine went on to write a humorous portrayal of her story in a book entitled *Not Now . . . I'm Having a No Hair Day!* Her book was nominated in two categories including "Best Motivational Book" of 1996 and "Best First Book" by the Books for a Better Life Awards. It won "Best Health Book of 1995/96" and "Best Illustrated Book" from the Midwest Independent Publishers Association. It won "Best Cover Design" and "Best Self Help/How-to Book" from the Mid-America Publishers Association. Her second book, especially for children, is entitled *Our Family Has Cancer, Too!* It won a prestigious Ben Franklin Award for Parenting (Family Issues/Child Care) from the Publishers Marketing Association. Her third book, *Inspiring Breakthrough Secrets to Live Your Dreams*, has been published by Aviva Publishing, Lake Placid, NY (December 2001).

Christine is a contributing author to *Chicken Soup for the Sur-*

vivor's Soul, *Chicken Soup for the Golfer's Soul*, *Chicken Soup for the Writer's Soul* and is featured in the books *The Courage to Laugh*, and *The Triumph of the Human Spirit—Real Cancer Survivors, Real Battles, Real Victories.*

Christine is currently president and chief executive officer of The Cancer Club®, a company designed to market humorous and helpful products internationally for people who have cancer. A dynamic speaker, she is currently touring on behalf of organizations world wide with her lectures on using humor and exercise to recover from chronic illness.

She serves as a spokesperson for HealthEast Care Systems and helped launch their new breast care center in May 2000. She also serves on the Board of Directors for the Minnesota Oncology Hematology Foundation.

She has been featured in *Better Homes & Gardens*, *MORE* magazine, *American Health*, *Today's Christian Woman*, *Golf Digest*, as well as *The Singapore Women's Weekly* and the *Hindu* in India. She was a 1998 "Hero Award" finalist for *Coping* magazine, and appeared on *CNN Live* in 1998 as "one of the world's leading authorities on the use of therapeutic humor." She also appeared on Lifetime Television Network's *New Attitudes* show and the *Leeza* Show.

Host of *The Christine Clifford Celebrity Golf Invitational*, a benefit for breast cancer research, Christine's inaugural event raised over $100,000, making it the most successful first-year event in the history of the American Cancer Society. Her annual event has raised over $600,000. She has received the Council of Excellence Award for income development from the American Cancer Society.

Christine is a member of the Minnesota Speakers Association, the National Speakers Association, the Association for Applied and Therapeutic Humor, and the National Association of Breast Cancer Organizations. She is listed in the International Who's Who of Professionals, International Who's Who of Entrepreneurs, and International Who's Who of Authors and Writers. She is also listed in *Contemporary Authors* and *2,000 Notable American Women*.

She lives with her husband, John, sons, Tim and Brooks, and dog, Sneakers, in Edina, Minnesota.

About the Illustrator

A native Minnesotan, **Jack Lindstrom** graduated with a B.F.A. from the Minneapolis College of Art and Design and operates F.A.B. Artists, Inc., an art studio in Minneapolis.

He specializes in humorous illustration for various print media—books, periodicals, and newspapers. For the past ten years he has collaborated with William Wells to produce a daily comic strip, *Bull 'N' Bears* for United Feature Syndicate. He is also a partner in Finkstrom Productions specializing in greeting cards and humorous calendars.

Jack is married to his high school sweetheart, receives unsolicited advice from two grown children and helps to spoil his three grandchildren whenever the opportunity presents itself . . . which is often.

About the Cancer Club®

A shared gift of laughter is a priceless gift to the spirit.

—CHRISTINE CLIFFORD

The Cancer Club®, based in Minneapolis, Minnesota, was created by Christine Clifford in 1995 in response to her experience with breast cancer. Christine, whose mother died of breast cancer at age forty-two, found that during her own treatment, family and friends were supportive, but they also were careful to avoid humorous conversation or topics around her.

Needing a lift, Christine began to search for signs of humor in herself and her predicament. She found them daily. The more she laughed, the stronger she grew, and The Cancer Club® was born.

The critically acclaimed Cancer Club® is the first organization to offer hope and support to cancer patients, their families, and friends through the healing power of humor. It serves as an international clearinghouse for people affected by cancer, offering inspirational gifts and providing information and resources through a quarterly newsletter.

Cancer Club® products include *Not Now . . . I'm Having A No Hair Day!*, Christine's story of her journey with cancer and the first book to address cancer from a humorous perspective. Her second book, entitled *Our Family Has Cancer, Too!*, was written especially for children. Other Cancer Club® items include video-tapes, PC software, Attitude pins, custom jewelry, coffee mugs, T-shirts, notepads, a special exercise video for women recovering from breast cancer surgery, and audiocassettes including Christine's lecture, "Laughter: A New Twist to the Old Illness of Cancer." The Cancer Club® also produces a quarterly newsletter.

Christine Clifford is president and chief executive officer of The Cancer Club®. As a member of the National Speakers Association, she lectures and tours on behalf of many organizations nationwide and is happy to share her story with you.

For more information about The Cancer Club®, call (952) 944-0639. Or write:

The Cancer Club®
6533 Limerick Drive
Edina, Minnesota 55439
Fax: (952) 941-1229
E-mail: Christine@cancerclub.com
www.cancerclub.com

Other Books by Christine Clifford

Not Now . . . I'm Having a No Hair Day!
Humor and Healing for People with Cancer
University of Minnesota Press. (June 1996) $9.95

In her straightforward style, forty-one-year-old, first-time author Christine Clifford paints a realistic picture of what it's like to discover cancer, undergo surgery, and endure radiation and chemotherapy treatments. But unlike most cancer patients, she manages to find humor in herself and her predicament.

Throughout the book, her moments of fear, uncertainty, love, and joy are captured by the gentle wit of illustrator Jack Lindstrom in sixty cartoons that reveal the vulnerability and strength of the human soul.

Whether you have cancer or know someone who does, Christine's story will touch your heart, make you laugh, and give you hope.

> *"Christine Clifford's* Not Now . . . I'm Having a No
> Hair Day! *is a wonderful book. Humor—that's the most*
> *important ingredient for facing the enemy-cancer."*
> —JULIE HARRIS, STAR OF STAGE, SCREEN, AND TELEVISION

This was the first book on the subject to offer hope to cancer victims, their families and friends through the healing power of humor.

Our Family Has Cancer, Too!
University of Minnesota Press. (October 1998) $6.95

When someone in your family gets cancer, find a way to go on living, laughing, playing and enjoying life to its fullest. Providing comfort through knowledge that "you are not alone," *Our Family Has Cancer, Too!* is an ideal gift for children ages five to fourteen whose families have been touched by cancer. In this eye-opening book, eleven-year-old Tim Clifford tells readers what it was like for him and his younger brother, Brooks, to support their mom while she was being treated for breast cancer.

Young people will appreciate the book's "open door" format, which encourages them to actively learn about their family's situation. A special "Questions to Ask" section following Tim's story invites kids to write down their questions for parents, doctors, teachers, and others. Additional worksheets inspire family members to draw and record their feelings for later discussion. The book also contains a glossary of the twenty-three most common words kids might hear when someone in their family gets cancer. Parents, too, gain valuable insight in learning how to talk about cancer more effectively with their kids. Powerful "Stop and Discuss" suggestions throughout the book encourage dialog between parents and children.

Throughout this book, the children's feelings of fear, uncertainty, hope, and love are poignantly depicted in eighteen illustrations of talking about cancer with family and friends. And remember, you are not alone: *Our Family Has Cancer, Too!*

To order an autographed copy of any of Christine's books today, call 1-800-586-9062 or visit www.cancerclub.com

Inspiring Breakthrough Secrets to Live Your Dreams
AVIVA Publishing, Lake Placid, NY (December 2001) $19.95

> "If you believe in yourself, your product, your service, or your cause, anything is possible."
> —CHRISTINE CLIFFORD

North America's most inspiring authorities in personal and professional transformation reveal secrets, insights, and strategies that will empower you to break through your limitations and live your dreams.

In her straightforward style, forty-eight-year-old author, professional speaker and president/CEO of The Cancer Club®, Christine Clifford believes adversity can be the stepping-stone to living your dream. In her chapter "The Blessings of Misfortune: Learn to Spin Straw into Gold," Christine will lead you through the steps that will help your dreams come true.

> "Everyone wants to have a breakthrough now. This master teacher has, at long last, congealed her genius in this book.

You can create phenomenal breakthroughs. Read it! Use it! Share it! And make your life a masterpiece."

—MARK VICTOR HANSON, CO-CREATOR,
#1 *NEW YORK TIMES* BEST-SELLING
CHICKEN SOUP FOR THE SOUL SERIES